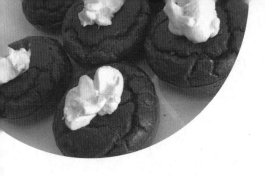

THE
KETO
SOLUTION

A Practical Guide for Living
Your Low-Carbohydrate Life

ANGELA DOUCETTE

T0017810

ACORNPRESS

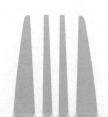

The Keto Solution: A Practical Guide for Living Your Low-Carbohydrate Life
ISBN 978-1-77366-046-2

Designed by Kenny Vail, Prevail Creative
Editing by Laurie Brinklow
Printed in Canada

The publisher acknowledges the support of the Government of Canada and the Province of Prince Edward Island for their support in our publishing efforts.

Library and Archives Canada Cataloguing in Publication

Title: The keto solution : a practical guide for living your
                low-carbohydrate life / Angela Doucette.

Names: Doucette, Angela, author.

Description: Includes index.

Identifiers: Canadiana (print) 2019014601X
                Canadiana (ebook) 20190146028
                ISBN 9781773660462 (softcover)
                ISBN 9781773660479 (PDF)

Subjects: LCSH: Ketogenic diet. | LCSH: Low-carbohydrate diet—Recipes.
LCSH: Reducing diets— Recipes. | LCGFT: Cookbooks.

Classification: LCC RM237.73 .D68 2020 | DDC 641.5/63837—dc23

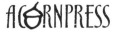
ACORNPRESS
P.O. Box 22024
Charlottetown, Prince Edward Island
C1A 9J2
acornpresscanada.com

"For all the educators, clinicians, and other health professionals in this field who are making a difference, one patient at a time."

AD

THE KETO SOLUTION

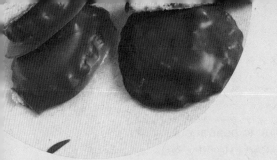

THE
KETO
SOLUTION

A Practical Guide for Living Your Low-Carbohydrate Life

Contents

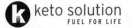

Foreword

As Angela's sister, I was one of the first to hear about it when she started following the Keto — or Low Carb, Healthy Fat — way of eating. I was apprehensive because it was counter to almost everything I had learned about "healthy" and "balanced" diets. It felt completely backward to me. How could eating things like cream cheese or bacon be okay, but apples and whole grains be off limits?

I couldn't ignore Angela's results, though.

In less than a year, she made an amazing transformation in her life. Not only did she lose weight, but her energy level, her mental health, and her cardiac risk factors all greatly improved. It was like she came alive in a whole new way. She was loving life, and didn't seem to be white-knuckling it to stay on plan. I was intrigued.

When I started following Keto, I quickly became aware of how much I had to learn. The first few times I went to the grocery store I felt lost because all of my former weight loss staples (rice cakes, fat-free yogurt, bananas, etc.) were suddenly off the table. I was lucky that I had Angela to walk me through the process, step by step. And now that you have your hands on this book, she will be able to guide you, too.

Angela has done countless hours of research, and has an unparalleled passion for helping others adopt this lifestyle. You are in good hands.

The sheer volume of information available online can be overwhelming and is often confusing. In this book, Angela distills the basic Keto principles into an easy-to-follow guide that will set you up for success. She shares her best tips and tricks, and a collection of favourite recipes developed by her and by the members of her Keto Solution community.

Although there are more Keto options becoming available at stores and restaurants, it's best if you can prepare a lot of your meals at home. Anyone who knows me knows that I hate to cook and bake. If you're like me, don't worry — you can do this! Keto meals can be extremely simple, such as bacon and eggs, or chicken and vegetables with butter. But if you're looking for greater variety or Keto-friendly alternatives to your favourite foods, the recipes in this book will certainly help.

The "Cheesecake on-the-Go" (p. 120) recipe is my personal favourite.

I had lost weight many times in the past using the low-calorie, low-fat approach. Even though I felt good about losing weight, I consistently felt deprived or hungry. Yet I believed this was the right way to shed the pounds. For me, the best part of switching to Keto was discovering the joy of FAT. It is the magic ingredient that will make you feel satisfied. When I am following Angela's plan, my stomach will growl if I haven't eaten in a while, but I never feel an intense, desperate urge to eat. There is a big difference.

If I could offer only one piece of advice, it would be this: don't try to go it alone. It's important to have people you can lean on, especially in the beginning as you learn about this new way of eating. Angela has created an amazing forum for this in her Facebook group. You can find it at: facebook.com/KetoSolution/groups. Members help one another, answer questions, and share ideas. If you haven't already, I encourage you to join this group for additional support.

I have seen people transform their lives through Angela's coaching. The power of food is undeniable; you just have to learn how to harness it. That's where this book comes in.

I wish you great success in your Keto journey!

~ Susan Howarth

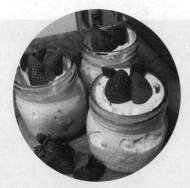

People are fed by the Food Industry, which pays no attention to health, and are treated by the Health Industry, which pays no attention to food.

— *Wendell Berry*

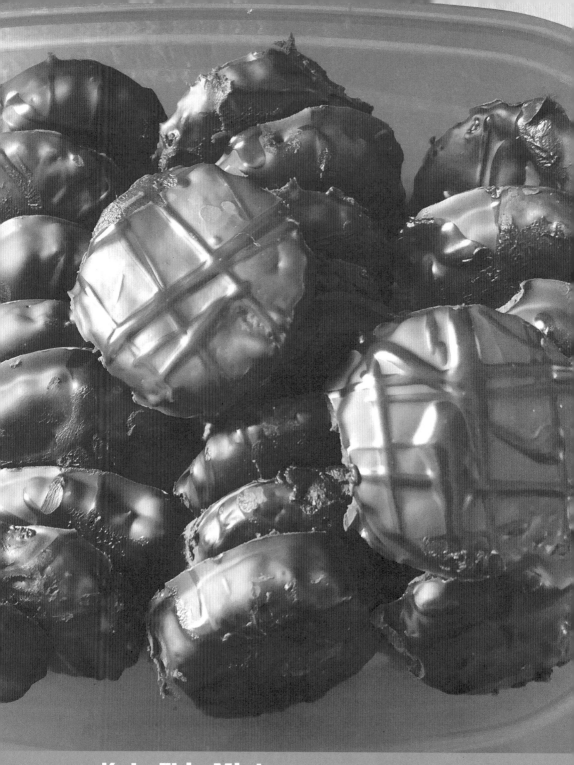

Keto Thin Mints > Desserts > Page 66

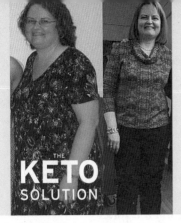

My Story / Introduction

We have all heard about the obesity and diabetes epidemics and there is no shortage of opinions on what to do about it. Most of the mainstream advice we hear is based on the "eat less/move more" philosophy, which is flawed for so many reasons. Our health system is strained under the weight of metabolic disease. More demand for services and limited resources make it feel like a losing battle to those on the front lines of health care.

According to 2019 data released by Diabetes Canada, 11 million Canadians live with diabetes or prediabetes and, costs have ballooned from $14 billion in 2008 to just under $30 billion. According to Statistics Canada, in 2018, 63.1% of Canadians 18 and older reported height and weight that classified them as overweight or obese. These are staggering statistics, but the good news is that there is hope.

By writing this book, I want to not only share personal success stories and recipes, I want to share information and tools to empower you to, in the words of Dr. Gary Fettke, "Make deposits into your health retirement"!

Like so many, I have a long history of battling my weight and my story might sound very familiar. In 2010, at the age of 40, I was seriously overweight and starting to show signs of metabolic disease. I had developed high blood pressure, had some concerning numbers in my cholesterol/lipid profile, and was about 50 pounds overweight. I lost my father in 1998, when he was 58, to heart disease, so I knew this was likely the path that I was on as well. I felt miserable and frustrated. I had tried so many weight loss and exercise programs over the years. I was 10 years old when I joined Weight Watchers for the first time! Nothing seemed to work long term. I did have some success counting calories and exercising, but after a while I would fall off the wagon and the weight would come back. I hated getting my picture taken, and when

I went clothes shopping, nothing ever seemed to fit or look right. The extra weight affected my confidence and I'm sure that influenced how I interacted with family and friends. I didn't want to participate in activities where I felt like people would be looking at me.

I always loved to cook and eat. Cooking special meals and treats for friends and family was a way for me to show affection. I was always conscious of trying to eat healthy and found it hard to understand why controlling my weight was so difficult when I thought I was "following the rules."

As a health professional, I felt embarrassed that I couldn't control my weight and needed medication. I felt defeated and felt that even if I tried again, I would likely fail just like all the other times. I also didn't feel I had any right to counsel patients on lifestyle changes when it was clear that I couldn't make any lasting changes myself.

My transformation goes back to May 2015. In my desperation for change, I decided to try a popular low-carb program using prepackaged foods along with weekly coaching. I did lose weight but was concerned about how I would maintain it. When I started doing further research, I came across the Keto way of eating (also known as LCHF, or Low Carb, Healthy Fat), which promoted using real food. When I changed my diet to Keto using natural, whole foods, I was finally able to shift the weight that had been such a source of frustration.

For the first time in my life, I felt like I had control and wasn't just a slave to my genes. With the weight loss came so many other positive changes in my life. I felt more confident, had more energy, and was having fun buying clothes in smaller sizes. I remember the first time I bought a Medium shirt. That felt like such a victory!

Most surprising was how it affected my health markers. My blood pressure decreased naturally, hs-CRP (an inflammatory marker) dropped significantly, and my lipid profile improved without medication. It's important to note that this was not just a result of losing weight. When I lost weight by counting calories, I did not see these same improvements in my health markers. As Dr. Gary Fettke says, "Once you see the benefits, you can't unsee them."

I remember thinking that this "discovery" would help others and decided to put together a public presentation on this way of eating in November 2015. It generated a lot of questions and interest. In early 2016, I started an in-person support group, created a Facebook group, and I built a website. I had no idea if anyone would be interested, but I needed a way to share what I was learning.

My following kept growing and the Facebook group that started out with a few friends and family has almost 2,000 members as of the publication of this book. The Keto Solution community group, which can be found through the Keto Solution Facebook Page, has a spirit of helping and supporting each other and I am so proud of what it has become. When someone is struggling or has a question, all they have to do is reach out and someone will respond with some helpful advice or some encouragement.

I have seen some amazing transformations over the last few years and am passionate about helping people find the path that works for them. When you can help someone lose significant amounts of weight and put their Type 2 Diabetes into remission, it is an incredible feeling. It is also rewarding to see those people pay it forward by helping and supporting others. I am fortunate to have friends, family, and co-workers who have been and continue to be so supportive and have been a big part of what Keto Solution has grown into. Whether helping on the admin team of the Facebook group, volunteering their time for educational events, or offering their advice and expertise, I am truly grateful.

This journey has not only changed my professional outlook, it has also given me hope for my own future. I believe I am doing all I can to minimize my risk of heart disease even with my strong family history. It has shown me that we are not a slave to our genes. We have more control than we think, and just need the knowledge and motivation to make the changes. I am most excited about helping people understand how powerful their food choices are in managing/preventing health issues, while decreasing dependence on medication.

If you have struggled with weight loss, and have tried other programs with little success, I put this guide together for you. I hope you will find the information and food ideas helpful to get you started on a new path.

Disclaimer

This guide does not provide individual medical advice and is not intended to diagnose, treat, cure, or prevent any disease.

Results may vary. There can be many different causes for being overweight or obese. Whether genetic or environmental, it should be noted that food intake, rates of metabolism, and levels of exercise and physical exertion vary from person to person. No individual result should be seen as typical.

The information, including but not limited to text, graphics, images, and other material, contained in this guide is for educational purposes only. The content is not intended in any way as a substitute for professional medical advice, diagnosis, or treatment. Always seek the advice of your physician or other qualified health care provider with any questions you may have regarding a medical condition or treatment and before undertaking a new health care regimen, and never disregard professional medical advice or delay in seeking it because of something you have read in this guide.

The nutritional information calculations were done using the online tool *MyFitnessPal*. Even though we have tried to provide accurate nutritional information, these figures should be considered estimates. Varying factors (such as product types or brands, natural fluctuations in fresh produce, substitutions, serving sizes, and the way ingredients are processed) change the effective nutritional information in any given recipe. Any change in ingredient will change the nutritional information, sometimes considerably. Different online calculators provide different results depending on their own nutrition-fact sources, databases, and algorithms. To obtain the most accurate representation of the nutritional information in a given recipe, please calculate the nutritional information with the actual ingredients and amounts used, using your preferred nutrition calculator.

What is Keto?

The word "Keto" can have many different interpretations and, with its current popularity, messages in the mainstream media and on the Internet can be confusing to navigate. The simple description of the ketogenic diet is restricting carbohydrates (sugar and starch) to 20–30 grams per day. This puts the body into a state of ketosis, which means the body uses mostly fat (both dietary and stored body fat) for fuel. Burning fat for fuel produces ketones, which most cells in the body can efficiently use as a fuel source. This is where the ketogenic diet, or Keto for short, gets its name.

It is important to note that ketosis is not the same as ketoacidosis, which occurs mainly in Type 1 Diabetics. It can also occur in Type 2 Diabetics who lose the ability to produce insulin. With a functioning pancreas and the ability to produce insulin, the body maintains ketone levels within a safe range.

After 2–4 weeks on the ketogenic diet, your body becomes fat adapted which means that fat becomes your primary energy source. Body fat stores (even if you are not overweight) provide a large reservoir of energy (we can store over 40,000 calories as fat versus approximately 2,000 calories from glucose/ sugar). Most people find once they are fat adapted, and become efficient at fat-burning, hunger goes away and it is easier to stretch the interval between eating times.

There are many different reasons people follow a ketogenic lifestyle. It is used to help control many chronic conditions such as obesity, diabetes, epilepsy, irritable bowel syndrome, and arthritis. It is a naturally anti-inflammatory way of eating.

Metabolic Flexibility

From an ancestral point of view, our bodies are designed to transition easily between sugar-burning and fat-burning. Our ancestors did not always have a steady supply of food, so the ability to use stored body fat for fuel and to produce glucose (sugar) in the liver (a process called gluconeogenesis) meant we could survive significant periods of time without food.

In our modern food environment, many of us have lost our metabolic flexibility, which means we become trapped in a constant need to fill up our glucose/sugar stores rather than tap into the energy in our stored body fat. Following the Keto way of eating allows you to switch into the fat-burning mode, which will set you up for weight loss success.

Have you been told that sugar/glucose is the body's preferred fuel? While it is true that the body will burn sugar first, another way to look at it is that the body looks at a high blood sugar level as toxic. The body wants to keep our blood sugar level within a tight range. At any given time, there is only about a teaspoon (4 grams) of sugar in the bloodstream. If there is enough fat and protein in the diet, there is actually no biological need for carbohydrates (sugar/starch).

Two-compartment Model

Dr. Jason Fung, a Toronto-based Nephrologist and founder of the Intensive Dietary Management Program, uses a refrigerator/freezer analogy for the two energy compartments, glucose and fat:

Glucose stores are easily accessible, like food in your refrigerator, but storage capacity is limited.

Fat stores are virtually unlimited, but they are more difficult to access. Just like food in the freezer in the basement, it takes more effort!

Why Calorie Restriction Doesn't Work Long Term for Weight Loss

A typical calorie-restricted diet focuses on portion control and limiting fat. Another common recommendation is eating small frequent meals. This eating pattern can result in weight loss but can also slow down your metabolism.

It all comes back to insulin. Eating frequently, or eating low-calorie foods that are high in carbohydrates, will keep insulin levels elevated, making it much harder to burn fat. When your body can't access its fat stores for energy, and on top of that you restrict your calories, the body will try to conserve energy by burning fewer calories when at rest. This will make weight loss much more difficult. When usual eating resumes, rebound weight gain happens relatively quickly and often exceeds the amount lost during the diet.

Insulin as the Fat-storing Hormone

Eating a low-fat/high-carb diet and eating too often makes managing insulin levels difficult which makes it difficult to control hunger. Insulin is also known as the fat-storing hormone. It is important to limit insulin spikes as much as possible and the two best ways of doing that are to keep carbohydrates low and to use time-restricted feeding to allow insulin levels to come down (also known as intermittent fasting). Those of us over a certain age will remember hearing "don't eat between meals." That was good advice! When insulin levels come down, our body can then access our fat stores for energy. With a steady flow of available energy, hunger decreases and going longer periods of time without eating becomes easier.

Our typical western diet does not promote lowering insulin levels with average carbohydrate intake between 200 and 300 grams per day and eating/snacking frequently.

Hyperinsulinemia

High insulin levels in the blood, or hyperinsulinemia, is essentially being Type 2 diabetic, and is associated with weight gain, high blood pressure, increased risk of heart disease/stroke, and Alzheimer's Disease.

We only diagnose diabetes when blood sugar levels start to go up, but Type 2 diabetes actually starts with high insulin levels. The body requires more and more insulin to keep the blood sugar within a safe range, and eventually the insulin doesn't do the job anymore and the blood sugar starts to go up.

Blood tests to measure insulin levels are not done routinely, but there are other signs and symptoms to be aware of. These include weight gain (especially around the waist), intense hunger (the "hangries"), signs of low blood sugar (shakiness, dizziness, headache), skin tags, fatty deposits around or on the eyelids, patches of dark skin in body folds/creases (typically under arms, groin area, or back of the neck), high triglyceride blood level, and low HDL blood level.

Adopting a Keto lifestyle keeps insulin levels low, which has been shown to not only be a very effective way to manage Type 2 diabetes, but can actually put this disease into remission. *Virta Health* in the US published data in 2019 showing that after one year on a medically supervised program using a ketogenic diet, 60% of study participants reversed Type 2 diabetes and 94% reduced or discontinued insulin. They also showed that even with a higher-fat diet, many saw improvements in risk factors for heart disease.

Cholesterol

This is probably the number one health concern with low-carb/high-fat diets. When reviewing your numbers with your healthcare provider, it is important to look at the big picture.

The total cholesterol number on its own is not a reliable marker of risk of heart disease. Generally, with a well-formulated low-carb diet, HDL (also known as the "good" cholesterol) goes up, triglycerides go down, and LDL (also known as the "bad" cholesterol) may go up, go down, or stay the same.

The most important number in your cholesterol profile is actually one you have to calculate yourself. If you take your triglyceride level and divide it by your HDL level, you will get your triglyceride to HDL ratio. If this number is lower than 1 (ideally 0.7 or less), that is a fairly reliable marker that you have a healthy metabolism and your risk of a cardiovascular event such as a heart attack or stroke is quite low.

It is also important to factor in the other risk factors for cardiovascular disease that improve such as weight loss and lowered blood pressure. There are many online calculators available to assess risk of a cardiovascular event. One resource is the Canadian Cardiovascular Society online forms and calculators.

Stop Fearing Fat

Our fear of fat can be traced back to the 1950s and a "link" that was observed between fat in the diet, cholesterol, and heart disease. This hypothesis was never proven in clinical trials, but ended up influencing dietary guidelines around the world starting in the late 70s. Not only was the hypothesis never proven, scientific data that did not support it was either ignored or not published at all in the rush to "solve" the post–Second World War increase in heart disease. In response to the scientists who actively campaigned to wait for more evidence before publishing the low-fat dietary guidelines, Senator George McGovern famously said in 1977, "Senators don't have the luxury that the research scientist does of waiting until every last shred of evidence is in." If you want to learn more about the history leading up to the first dietary guidelines, published in 1980, I recommend the movie *Fathead* on YouTube or *Fat: A Documentary*.

Fat in the diet is important for many different functions including absorption of fat-soluble vitamins (A, D, E, and K), immune function, maintaining healthy skin and hair, and regulating body temperature, among others. On top of that, it makes our food taste better and keeps us full longer.

It is important to distinguish between different fats. Sticking to natural fat (such as butter, olive oil, coconut oil, cheese/full-fat dairy products, fatty fish, fatty cuts of meat) is preferable to manufactured vegetable oils, shortening, or margarine. These industrial products can promote inflammation and do not provide any nutritive value. Many people worry about increasing intake of animal fat and/or saturated fat in the diet. When the refined sugars, grains, starches, and processed/junk foods are eliminated, there is no evidence that I am aware of that animal fat intake is a concern.

Contrary to many diet apps and calculators, there is no target required for fat intake. The key is to use enough to enjoy your food and to control your appetite. There is no need to fear fat, but also no need to try to eat a certain amount. It is true that eating too much fat can stall weight loss. If you are not getting the results you are hoping for, cutting back a bit on the fat can be a useful strategy.

Is Keto Sustainable?

This question comes up a lot and is a common criticism of the low-carbohydrate way of eating. However, this eating pattern is easier to stick to than low-fat/low-calorie diets because you can eat delicious food until you are satisfied. When hunger decreases, it is naturally easier to eat less and not feel deprived. Many people who adopt a low-carb lifestyle never go back to their old eating patterns once they see the benefits.

There are many reasons why people may fall back into old habits such as food addiction, stress, hormonal imbalances, social pressures, or time constraints. It can happen to the best of us, but what brings people back is how much better they feel on a low-carb diet. For many, the treats are not worth the price. For those who have put their Type 2 diabetes into remission using carbohydrate restriction, there is extra motivation to keep going and avoid restarting medications to control blood sugar.

A good support system is also an important component for maintaining a low-carb/Keto lifestyle. Whether that support comes from family and friends, an online or in-person support group, your healthcare team, or a combination of these, it can make it much easier to keep going. Finding out what works for others, sharing recipes, and helping each other through the struggles of everyday life can make all the difference.

Basic Rules

1. Cut out processed foods (e.g. cereal, granola bars, chips, crackers, packaged snack foods, vegetable/seed oils, margarine).
2. Cut out sugar and starch (e.g. bread, potatoes, pasta, rice).
3. Choose natural fats and avoid margarine and industrial seed oils (e.g. canola, soy, corn).
4. Eat a variety of non-starchy vegetables (e.g. broccoli, cauliflower, peppers, cucumber, cabbage, turnip, zucchini).
5. Choose full-fat dairy products.
6. Choose your carbohydrate limit (total, not net): under 20 g for keto, 20–50 g for low-carb, 50–100 g for liberal low-carb.
7. Limit fruit to berries.
8. Eat when you are hungry, and stop when you are satisfied.
9. Stick to no-calorie drinks such as water, coffee, or tea; no juice or milk.
10. Avoid eating between meals and attempt to eat all your meals within an 8-hour window during the day.

What to Expect in the Beginning

If this way of eating is new to you, and your body is used to only burning sugar/glucose for energy, it can take some time for your body to adjust and become fat-adapted. Your cells need different machinery to get fired up to use fat for fuel. During the transition, you may experience headaches, fatigue, irritability, dizziness, and generally not feeling well. This is often referred to as the "Keto Flu." Not everyone will experience this and it may last anywhere from a few days to a few weeks. Be patient, and don't give up. Think of it as a sign that something important is happening in your body. Once your metabolism has made the switch, you will feel much better. A lot of people describe a feeling of mental clarity and alertness that they have never experienced before.

When you are fat-adapted and follow a Keto way of eating, your blood sugar will stabilize and you will no longer have the roller-coaster highs and lows. When blood sugar crashes, it triggers hunger, cravings, and can also lead to that "hangry" feeling of irritability and an intense need to eat.

Here you can see the difference in blood sugar levels over a few days following standard nutritional advice versus low-carb:

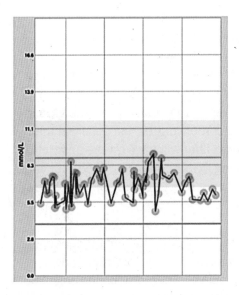 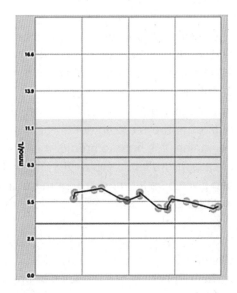

Graphs courtesy of Jill Sabean, Keto Solution Admin

Some strategies that can help minimize the unpleasant effects include staying hydrated and increasing salt intake. When you cut carbohydrates, and your insulin level drops, this signals your kidneys to release salt and water, so it is important to replace it. If you don't see any improvement, consult your healthcare provider since there might be more going on that requires investigation.

Macros

When you hear the term "macros," this is referring to the macronutrients: carbohydrates, protein, and fat. Macro recommendations are often made in percentages, which is not ideal. Each macronutrient should be looked at separately and calculated for each individual depending on what your goals are.

The level of carbohydrates should be chosen first. To follow a very low-carbohydrate/ketogenic diet, total carbohydrates have to be limited to around 20–30 grams per day. To follow a more liberal/low-carbohydrate diet, you can bump up the carbohydrates to 50–100 grams per day. Carbohydrates can be tracked as "total" or "net." Net carbohydrates are the total minus the grams of fiber. I always recommend tracking total carbohydrates, especially in the beginning. It is hard to predict the effect that fiber will have on the absorption of carbohydrates so you might end up taking in more than intended. Net carbs can give you a bit more freedom but it can be a bit misleading and may slow weight loss.

It is important to know what your protein requirements are. For most people, this is 0.6–1 gram per pound of lean body mass. This requirement may be higher depending on your level of physical activity. There are online calculators available to estimate your amount of lean body mass (the weight of your body minus body fat). For example, if your lean body mass is around 100 pounds, you would need 60–100 grams of protein. Proteins are the main building blocks for your body and are required for building/maintaining muscle, tendons, organs, and hormones. Protein is the most important macro to focus on since there is a target to meet.

As mentioned earlier, there is no minimum requirement for fat intake. If fat loss is your goal, backing off on the fat in the diet encourages your body to burn stored body fat for energy. When the ketogenic diet is described as being 70% fat, that doesn't mean you have to eat it all. What is burned from body fat is included in that 70%.

Tracking food using an online calculator or app is helpful in the beginning to get an idea of what food choices will meet your carbohydrate and protein goals. Most people don't have to use them forever. Once you are in a routine and getting the results you are looking for, tracking all the time won't usually be necessary. Just remember to ignore the fat recommendations.

Does It Matter When I Eat?

The short answer is yes, it does matter when you eat. Eating earlier in the day may be more in tune with our natural circadian rhythm and be more in line with our genetics. Having periods of time without food allows insulin levels to come down and encourages fat-burning. While some individuals may find better results with intermittent fasting, it is not required for weight loss. When you are used to burning fat for energy, and hunger decreases, intermittent fasting occurs naturally if you only eat when hungry.

There are many different fasting schedules including 16:8 (only eating during an 8-hour window each day), 24, 36, 48, or 72-hour fasts occasionally, or OMAD (one meal a day). Most people will concentrate on food choices at first and incorporate time-restricted feeding or intermittent fasting later. Too many changes at once can be overwhelming.

Two of the biggest myths around feeding schedules are "Breakfast is the most important meal of the day" and "You should eat small frequent meals to keep your metabolism up." When you look at the word "breakfast," it is just when you break your overnight fast. You can decide what time of day that is! If you eat 5–6 times a day, you don't give your insulin level a chance to come down and it makes losing weight more difficult. To lose weight following that eating pattern, you have to really restrict calories. If you only eat once or twice a day and restrict carbohydrates, you can tolerate higher-calorie meals, which makes eating much more enjoyable.

Exercise

Physical activity is important for overall health, but you can make significant improvements by food choices alone. For many, weight loss and improved energy naturally leads to more activity. When first starting the Keto way of eating, intense exercise is not advisable until you are efficient at burning fat for energy. During the transition period from a "sugar burner" to a "fat burner," your energy level will likely drop until you become fat-adapted. Exercise also generally causes an increased appetite, which may actually hinder weight loss. Incorporate more activity as your energy level increases. There are many benefits to exercise, but it is not very effective as a method to lose weight.

Shopping and Cooking Tips

Getting back to cooking at home is a big part of this way of eating. The best way to know what you are eating is to make it yourself. I know this does not sound appealing to many who are not crazy about spending time in the kitchen, but you really can make low-carb cooking simple and easy with just a bit of planning.

Have your list of staples and keep your kitchen well-stocked so meals can be put together in a pinch. Make your grocery list and stick to it. If online grocery ordering and pickup is available where you live, that can really save time — and you will also avoid the temptations of the grocery store, especially at the checkout. If you do shop in the store, stick to the perimeter as much as possible: for produce, meat, eggs, dairy, and frozen vegetables.

Plan what you will eat for the week. This usually means only 3–4 meals if you make enough for leftovers. It is also a great idea to freeze some prepared meals to grab when you need something quick. Cooking extra meat and preparing veggies ahead of time makes throwing together lunches quick and easy.

Keep just enough variety so you don't get bored, but don't overcomplicate it either. For example, you don't have to have bacon and eggs every morning. Make a quiche and freeze it in portions, make low-carb pancakes, have plain yogurt with some berries and a bit of protein powder sweetened with stevia. Once you get into a routine, and have a rotation of your favourites, it will get easier!

Substitutions

Pasta/Noodles	Zucchini
Rice	Cauliflower Rice or Grated Zucchini
Wheat Flour	Coconut Flour/Almond Flour (amounts vary)
Taco Shells/Tortillas	Raw Cabbage Leaf/Lettuce Wrap
Pop	Sparkling Water
Sugar	Erythritol/Stevia
Potatoes	Cauliflower or Daikon Radish
Margarine/Shortening	Butter
Vegetable Oil	Coconut Oil/Olive Oil
Sweet Potato	Pumpkin + Riced Cauliflower
Pizza Crust	Cheese/Egg/Almond Flour Crust (Fathead)
Cereal	Sugar-free/Grain Free Granola
Croutons	Parmesan Crisps
Spaghetti	Spaghetti Squash
French Fries	Turnip Fries
Macaroni	Cauliflower
Wheat Flour as Thickener (Soups/Gravy)	Xanthan Gum or Glucomannan (amounts vary)

Cheat Days

This is a controversial subject and there are many different opinions on cheat days. They can be a slippery slope since hunger and cravings can be triggered. It can take anywhere from a few days to a couple of weeks to get back on track. Pay attention to how you feel after a high-carb indulgence. You may feel sluggish and experience "brain fog," especially if you've been following Keto for any length of time. Many people don't find the cheat days worth it. Over time, your tastes will change and the sugar/starch won't be so appealing. In my experience, the cheats happen more for social or emotional reasons rather than missing the actual food.

If you want to treat yourself without going overboard, try reaching for a small serving of Chapman's No Sugar Added ice cream, or a Keto dessert such as "Cheesecake on-the-Go" with some berries and/or grain-free granola.

Eating Out

Eating out can be challenging, especially in the beginning, but for the most part, restaurants are very accommodating if you know what to ask for. Even at a fast food restaurant, there are lettuce bun options for burgers and, of course, salads.

Sometimes, you can only make the best choice you can. Focusing on protein and vegetables will get you most of the way there. Ask for extra vegetables instead of potatoes/pasta/rice, and skip the bread.

Sample Meal Plan

Breakfast at 9AM, Lunch at Noon, Snack at 3PM (if needed), Dinner at 5PM
12–18 hours between Dinner and Breakfast on most days

Breakfast

	Calories kcal	Carbs g	Fat g	Protein g	Sodium mg	Fiber g
Coffee - Brewed from grounds, 1 cup (8 fl oz)	2	0	0	0	5	0
Cream 18% - Cream 18%, 2 tbsp	60	2	5	1	10	0
Pc - Skyr Plain Yogurt 4 %, 175 g	170	8	7	19	65	0
kaizen - whey protein , 1 scoop	150	3	1	35	65	1
Superstore - Frozen Berries, 0.5 cup (140g)	40	9	0	1	0	3
Ditch the Carbs - Grain-free Granola, 40 g	317	9	29	6	0	5
Add Food | Quick Tools	739	31	42	62	145	9

Lunch

	Calories	Carbs	Fat	Protein	Sodium	Fiber
Superstore - Roast Chicken, 3 ounce	170	0	10	20	281	0
Homemade - Olive Oil and Apple Cider Vinegar Dressing, 2 Tbsp	122	1	14	0	0	0
Generic - Tossed Salad With Peppers and Cucumbers, 1 cup	75	11	4	1	2	4
Add Food | Quick Tools	367	12	28	21	283	4

Dinner

	Calories	Carbs	Fat	Protein	Sodium	Fiber
Crack Slaw, 1 serving(s)	312	7	19	26	985	3
Add Food | Quick Tools	312	7	19	26	985	3

Snacks

Add Food \| Quick Tools

Totals	1,418	50	89	109	1,413	16

My Kitchen Staples

- Eggs
- Cheese (cheddar, mozzarella, fresh parmesan)
- Full Fat Cream Cheese
- Full Fat Sour Cream
- Whipping Cream
- Mayonnaise: Hellman's Olive Oil
- Mustard
- Non-starchy Vegetables, fresh or frozen (broccoli, cauliflower, turnip, cucumber peppers, onions, zucchini, spaghetti squash, lettuce/greens)
- Meats (bacon, chicken, ground beef)
- Plain Yogurt (5–10% fat)
- Frozen Avocado Chunks (for smoothies)
- Frozen Berries
- Kalamata Olives
- No Sugar Added Syrup (e.g., Mrs. Butterworth's)
- No Sugar Added Vanilla Ice Cream (occasional treat)
- Nuts/Seeds (almonds, pecans, sunflower seeds, pumpkin seeds)
- Cocoa
- Parmesan Crisps — Costco
- Unsweetened Coconut
- Coconut Oil — Costco
- Olive Oil — Costco
- Bragg Organic Apple Cider Vinegar — Bulk Barn
- Spice Mixes (Onion/Chive. Italian/Pizza, Greek, Ranch, Montreal Steak, Montreal Chicken, Southwest/Taco)
- Minced Garlic
- Sea Salt — Costco
- Almond Flour — Bulk Barn or Costco
- Coconut Flour — Bulk Barn
- Erythritol/Stevia Sweetener — Bulk Barn
- Pro Granola — Simply for Life Market or Amazon or Well.ca
- Krisda Chocolate Chips
- Sparkling Water
- Stur Brand Sugar Free Water Flavouring
- Lemon Juice

My Favourite Local Businesses

When I first started Keto, it could be quite challenging to find food choices that fit my eating plan. Thankfully, it is much easier today. Many restaurants and businesses are more aware of Keto due to customer demand. Here is my list of favourites:

- **Superstore** — shopping online saves time and avoids temptations
- **Riverview Country Market** — local meat, cheese, preserves and produce as well as Keto-friendly frozen foods (fat bombs, pizza, baked goods)
- **Price Mart** — carries many Costco items such as nuts, almond flour, parmesan crisps, olive oil, coconut oil
- **Bulk Barn** — nuts, seeds, organic apple cider vinegar, almond flour, coconut flour, erythritol/stevia sweetener
- **Simply for Life Market** — snack bars, granola, crackers, sauces, ready-made meals
- **Maid Marian's Diner** — Keto choices include bacon/eggs, steak sandwich without the bun with Caesar salad
- **Papa Joe's** — Keto choices include Mediterranean salad with chicken (skip the bread and tortilla crisps), butter chicken (skip the rice), burgers without the bun and salad instead of fries

THE KETO SOLUTION

BREAKFAST

90-second Bread

1 serving

Prep/total time: 5 mins

Ingredients
1/3 cup almond flour
1 egg
1 tbsp butter
1 tbsp baking powder
1/2 tbsp garlic powder
1/2 tbsp dill seed (optional)

Directions
- Melt butter in a 4-6-inch microwave-safe dish
- Whisk in remaining ingredients, and heat on high 90 secs
- Fry or toast to crisp up

Nutritional Information per serving
387 calories
33 g fat
8 g carbohydrates
4 g fiber
14 g protein

Avocado Smoothie

1 serving

Prep/total time: 5 mins

Ingredients
1/2 cup frozen avocado chunks
1/4 cup frozen berries
1 scoop vanilla protein powder
(sweetened with Stevia)
1 tbsp cocoa powder
1 cup water
1/2 cup unsweetened coconut milk

Directions
- Blend until smooth

Nutritional Information per serving
298 calories
20 g carbohydrates
7 g fiber
24 g protein
17 g fat

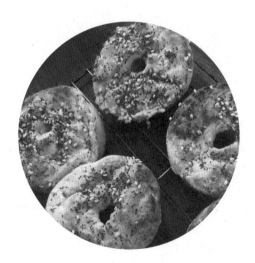

Bagels

6 bagels

Prep time: 5 mins
Total time: 20 mins

Ingredients
1/2 cup coconut flour OR 3/4 cup
almond flour
1 tbsp baking powder
2 1/2 cups shredded cheese
2 oz cream cheese
2 eggs, beaten
sesame seeds for topping

Directions
- Preheat oven to 400° F
- In a bowl stir together flour and
  baking powder; set aside
- In a separate bowl, heat the
  shredded cheese and cream
  cheese for 2 mins, stirring halfway
  through; mix well
- Stir the flour mix and eggs into the
  cheeses and mix well (you can chill
  the dough at this point to make it
  easier to work with)
- Divide dough into 6 equal parts
  and roll into logs; press ends
  together to form bagels
- Sprinkle with sesame seeds
- Bake for 10-14 mins until golden

Nutritional Information per bagel
271 calories
19 g fat
6 g carbohydrates
3.6 g fiber
14 g protein

Bulletproof Hot Cocoa

1 serving

Prep/total time: 5 mins

Ingredients
1 1/4 cups water OR almond milk OR
coconut milk
1 1/2 tbsp cocoa powder
1/2-1 tbsp sweetener such as
erythritol
2 tbsp heavy whipping cream
1/4 tsp vanilla extract
1 tbsp butter OR coconut oil OR MCT
oil (optional)

Directions
- Heat water/milk until hot
- Add cocoa powder, sweetener,
  vanilla extract, and optional add-ins

Nutritional Information per serving
225 calories
23 g fat
7 g carbohydrates
3 g fiber
2 g protein

Blueberry/ Cranberry Muffins

12 muffins

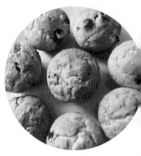

Prep time: 10 mins
Total time: 30 mins

Ingredients
2 1/2 cups almond flour
1/2 cup Swerve
1 1/2 tsp baking powder
1/2 tsp sea salt (optional, but recommended)
1/3 cup coconut oil (measured solid, then melted; can also use butter)
1/3 cup unsweetened almond milk
3 large egg
1/2 tsp vanilla extract
3/4 cup blueberries OR cranberries

Directions
- Preheat the oven to 350° F; line a muffin pan with 12 silicone or parchment paper muffin liners
- In a large bowl stir together the almond flour, erythritol, baking powder, and sea salt
- Mix in the melted coconut oil, almond milk, eggs, and vanilla extract; fold in the blueberries
- Distribute the batter evenly among the muffin cups
- Bake for about 20 mins, until the top is golden, and an inserted toothpick comes out clean

Nutritional Information per muffin
217 calories
19 g fat
6 g carbohydrates
3 g fiber
7 g protein

Breakfast Biscuits

1 serving

Prep/total time: 5 mins

Ingredients
1 tbsp butter
1 tbsp coconut flour
1 tbsp sour cream
1 egg
1/8 tsp baking powder

Directions
- Melt butter in mug for 30 secs
- Add coconut flour, sour cream, egg, and baking powder; mix well to get dough texture
- Microwave mug for 90 secs
- Serve with sugar-free jam (such as Smuckers sugar-free raspberry)

Nutritional Information per serving
228 calories
19 g fat
5 g carbohydrates
2.5 g fiber
7.5 g protein

Buffalo Blue Cheese Omelette

1 serving

Prep time: 5 mins
Total time: 10 mins

Ingredients
Omelette
2 eggs
1 tbsp water
1 tbsp butter for frying

Filling
1 oz cream cheese
1/2-1 tbsp blue cheese dressing
1 1/2 tsp hot sauce

Directions
- Mix eggs and water together; fry in butter
- Place filling ingredients in a small bowl and heat slightly and stir together
- Add filling to one side of the omelette and cover over with the other side of the egg
- Cover for 2 mins

Nutritional Information per serving
376 calories
33 g fat
3.7 g carbohydrates
1.5 g fiber
15.9 g protein

Chocolate Peanut Butter Protein Shake

1 serving

Prep/total time: 5 mins

Ingredients
2 tbsp cream cheese
1 cup unsweetened vanilla cashew OR almond milk
1 tbsp natural peanut butter (no sugar or salt)
1 scoop Stevia-sweetened chocolate protein powder
1/2 tsp vanilla
ice

Directions
- Blend all ingredients together in blender

NOTE: An option is to switch out peanut butter and add instant coffee or espresso powder for a mocha protein shake

Nutritional Information per serving
334 calories
19.5 g fat
7.7 g carbohydrates
4 g fiber
32.7 g protein

Cream Cheese Pancakes

6 pancakes

Prep time: 5 mins
Total time: 15 mins

Ingredients
4 oz cream cheese, softened
4 eggs
1 tsp vanilla extract
1 tbsp erythritol/Stevia mix
4 tbsp coconut flour
2 tsp baking powder
1 tbsp butter (for frying)

Directions:
- Cream eggs and cream cheese and vanilla
- Add other ingredients and mix until smooth
- Melt butter in frying pan and fry pancakes until golden brown and cooked through

Nutritional Information per pancake
135 calories
10 g fat
4.5 g carbohydrates
1.5 g fiber
6 g protein

Egg and Cheese Crustless Quiche

6 servings

Prep time: 5 mins
Total time: 50 mins

Ingredients
6 eggs
4 oz shredded cheese, divided
2 oz cream cheese
6 tbsp butter, melted
salt and pepper to taste

NOTE: Extra toppings, such as ham, bacon, veggies, or other spices, are not reflected in nutritional information

Directions
- Add half the cheese to a casserole dish
- Add eggs and cream cheese to a food processor/blender and mix
- Slowly add melted butter to the egg and cream cheese
- Pour egg mixture over cheese in dish and top with remaining cheese; top with chives or parsley
- Bake at 325° F for 40-45 mins

Nutritional Information
per serving
220 calories
20 g fat
1.5 g carbohydrates
0 g fiber
9 g protein

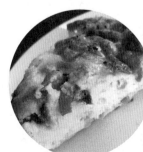

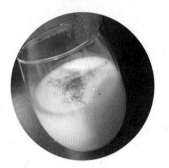

Fat Milkshake

1 serving

Prep/total time: 5 mins

Ingredients
1 tbsp cream cheese
1 egg
1 tsp vanilla extract
1 tbsp MCT oil OR coconut oil
1/4 cup heavy whipping cream
3-4 ice cubes

Directions
- Blend all ingredients together in blender

Nutritional Information per serving
433 calories
43 g fat
2 g carbohydrates
0 g fiber
7 g protein

Feta and Cream Cheese Quiche

6 servings

Prep time: 15 mins
Total time: 60 mins

Crust
3/4 cup almond flour
1 egg
1 tbsp coconut flour
salt and pepper

Crust directions
- Press crust into 8x8" greased glass dish and bake at 350° F for 8-10 mins

Filling
1 tbsp butter
1/2 red pepper, diced
1/2 cup onion, chopped
2 cups fresh spinach
6 eggs
2 tbsp 18% cream
1/2 cup crumbled feta cheese
4 oz (half-package) cream cheese cut into chunks

Filling Directions
- Sauté red pepper and onion in butter; add spinach and cook until wilted
- Spread veggies over cooked crust
- Mix together eggs, cream, feta cheese, and cream cheese
- Pour mixture over veggies
- Bake at 350° F for 40-50 mins until cooked through

Nutritional Information per serving
280 calories
25.5 g fat
7.5 g carbohydrates
2.5 g fiber
14 g protein

Flax Bagels

4 bagels

Prep time: 5 mins
Total time: 20 mins

Ingredients
1/2 cup ground flax seed
2 tbsp cream cheese
1 1/2 cups shredded mozzarella
cheese
1 egg
everything bagel seasoning to top

Directions
- Preheat oven to 400° F
- Melt cheeses together in microwave
- Mix egg and flax seed together then
  add in melted cheeses
- Mix until dough forms
- Place 4 rolled balls of dough on
  lined baking sheet, press down and
  poke holes in the centres
- Sprinkle with seasoning
- Bake 15 mins

Nutritional Information per bagel
310 calories
24 g fat
9.8 g carbohydrates
8 g fiber
17.6 g protein

French Toast Sticks

14 servings of 2 sticks

Prep time: 5 mins
Total time: 15 mins

Ingredients
French toast sticks
2 tbsp olive oil OR butter
4 eggs
3/4 cup almond flour
1 tbsp baking powder
1 tbsp maple extract

Coating
2 eggs
1/8 cup heavy whipping cream
1 tbsp cinnamon
1 tbsp vanilla

Directions
- Whisk all the French toast stick
  ingredients together
- Grease a microwavable bowl; heat the
  mixture 3-4 mins or until firm
- Cut into sticks
- Mix coating ingredients in a bowl; dip sticks
- Heat oil/butter in a skillet and cook
  sticks 1 min per side
- Serve with butter and sugar-free maple
  syrup and whipped cream if desired

NOTE: Can be stored in the refrigerator
and reheated

Nutritional Information per serving
(2 sticks)
210 calories
16 g fat
5.8 g carbohydrates
3.4 g fiber
6.6 g protein

Granola Bars
10 servings

Prep time: 10 mins
Total time: 30 mins

Ingredients
1/2 cup almond butter
1/4 cup coconut oil
2 tsp vanilla
1/3 cup Swerve
1/2 cup sliced almonds
1/3 cup ground flax seed
1 tbsp chia seeds
1/3 cup pumpkin seeds
1/4 cup unsweetened shredded coconut
1 tsp cinnamon
2 oz sugar-free chocolate, melted, for drizzling

Directions
- In a bowl, melt almond butter, coconut oil, and vanilla in the microwave 30 secs; repeat until fully melted
- Add sweetener and heat another 30 secs and mix
- In another bowl mix together all dry ingredients; add the wet mixture and fully incorporate
- Spread mixture into a parchment-paper-lined 9x5" pan and freeze 20 mins
- Remove and drizzle with chocolate and sliced almonds

Nutritional Information per serving
350 calories
30 g fat
12 g carbohydrates
9 g fiber
9.8 g protein

Green Smoothie
1 serving

Prep/total time: 5 mins

Ingredients
2 cups spinach
2 tbsp Stevia OR sweetener of choice
1/2 avocado, pitted and chopped
1 cup unsweetened almond milk
1 1/2 cups ice

Directions
- Put the spinach in a blender and process until smooth
- Add milk and other ingredients, and blend on high to make a smooth mixture
- Garnish with crushed almonds and serve

Nutritional Information per serving
161 calories
13 g fat
9 g carbohydrates
6.3 g fiber
4.2 g protein

Golden Keto Bread
20 slices

Prep time: 10 mins
Total time: 60 mins

Ingredients
6 eggs
1 block cream cheese, softened
6 tbsp olive oil
1 1/2 cups almond flour
3 tbsp psyllium husk powder
1 tsp salt
2 tsp baking powder

Directions
- Preheat oven to 350° F
- Beat the egg
- Add cream cheese and olive oil
- Add all dry ingredients
- Blend well
- Pour into greased loaf pan
- Bake 45 mins

Nutritional Information per slice
148 calories
13.3 g fat
3.1 g carbohydrates
2.4 g fiber
4.5 g protein

Mock Oatmeal
1 serving

Prep time: 2 mins
Total time: 5 mins

Ingredients
2 tbsp coconut flour
4 tbsp unsweetened coconut, shredded
1 tbsp Swerve
3/4 cup almond OR coconut milk, unsweetened
1 tbsp almond butter OR natural peanut butter

Directions
- Combine all ingredients together in a saucepan
- Heat to a simmer then bring to a boil, then lower heat and simmer 2-3 mins until thickened
- Remove from heat when you reach desired consistency
- Serve with berries or favourite toppings
- Optional add-ins: cinnamon, nutmeg, sugar-free maple syrup/ brown sugar

Nutritional Information per serving
330 calories
27 g fat
18 g carbohydrates
13 g fiber
8 g protein

No-oatmeal
1 serving

Prep/total time: 5 mins

Ingredients
1 cup water
2 tbsp chia seeds
2 tbsp ground flax seeds
2 tbsp butter
2 tbsp heavy whipping cream
2 tbsp natural/no sugar added
peanut butter (optional)

Directions
- Boil water on stovetop
- Add chia and flax seeds; turn down
  heat until it thickens, about 1-2
  mins
- Pour into a bowl; add butter, heavy
  cream, and peanut butter, and mix
- Additional toppings: cinnamon,
  berries, nutmeg

Nutritional Information per serving
352 calories
30.5 g fat
10 g carbohydrates
8 g fiber
7.4 g protein

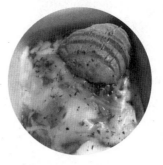

Pizza Eggs
1 serving

Prep time: 5 mins
Total time: 10 mins

Ingredients
2 eggs
2 tbsp pizza sauce (low-sugar)
2 slices pepperoni, cut into quarters
(8 small pieces)
2 oz cheese

Directions
- In a microwave-safe dish precook
  the eggs roughly 2 mins
- Add your sauce, cheese, and
  pepperoni and place back in
  microwave an additional 2 mins
- Garnish with sprinkle of parsley or
  oregano
- Depending on your egg preference
  you can lessen or add more
  cooking time

Nutritional Information per serving
178 calories
11.9 g fat
3.2 g carbohydrates
0.5 g fiber
13.8 g protein

Power Smoothie

1 serving

Prep/total time: 5 mins

Ingredients
1 cup spinach
4 walnuts
4 raspberries
1 tsp chia seeds
1 cup almond milk (unsweetened)
2 tbsp heavy cream
1 tbsp coconut oil, melted, OR MCT oil
2 ice cubes

Directions
- Put all the ingredients in a blender, except coconut oil, and mix until smooth
- Pour into a tall glass, and add the coconut oil; stir with spoon to mix the oil

Nutritional Information per serving
295 calories
29 g fat
4.4 g carbohydrates
2.7 g fiber
3.3 g protein

Salted Caramel Custards

2 Servings

Prep time: 5 mins
Total time: 1 1/2 hrs

Ingredients
Custard
2 eggs
2 oz cream cheese
1 cup water
1 1/2 tbsp Swerve sweetener
1 1/2 tsp caramel extract

Sauce
2 tbsp butter
2 tbsp Swerve
1/2 tsp caramel extract

Directions
- Preheat oven to 325° F
- Combine all ingredients in a blender and mix well
- Pour into greased 6 oz ramekin dishes
- Place dishes onto baking sheet and fill with water until halfway up the ramekin dish
- Bake for 30 mins
- Remove and let chill 1 hr
- Once chilled, melt sauce ingredients for 30 secs in microwave; divide into two portions and pour over custards before serving

Nutritional Information per serving
272 calories
26.2 g fat
5.5 g carbohydrates
0 g fiber
8 g protein

Sausage Biscuits
24 servings

Prep time: 10 mins
Total time: 50 mins

Ingredients
1 LB bulk sausage meat
2 tbsp butter, melted
4 eggs
3/4 cup fresh shredded Parmesan cheese
1 cup almond flour

Directions
-Mix all ingredients
-Shape into 24 patties
-Bake at 350° F for 30-40 mins until cooked through

Nutritional Information per serving
110 calories
9 g fat
1.7 g carbohydrates
0.5 g fiber
5.7 g protein

Shakshuka
6 servings

Prep time: 10 mins
Total time: 30 mins

Ingredients
1 medium onion, diced
1 red pepper, seeded and diced
4 garlic cloves, finely chopped
2 tsp paprika
1 tsp cumin
1/4 tsp chili powder
1 can whole peeled tomatoes (28 OZ)
6 eggs
salt and pepper to taste

Directions
- Heat a couple tablespoons of olive oil in a pan over medium heat; add red pepper and onion and cook about 5 mins or until the onions become translucent
- Add garlic and spices and cook for another minute or so
- Pour canned tomatoes and juice into the pan and break down the tomatoes with spatula; add salt and pepper and bring to a simmer
- Using spatula or a spoon, make wells in the sauce and add eggs into each well
- Cover and cook 5-8 mins or until eggs are cooked to your liking
- Garnish with fresh cilantro and parsley (optional)

more...

Continued...

NOTE: This recipe is very versatile as the ingredients and spices can all be changed to your liking. For example, you could add spinach, mushrooms, or other vegetables of your preference.

Nutritional Information per serving
122 calories
5 g fat
9.5 g carbohydrates
2 g fiber
8 g protein

Snickerdoodle Pancakes
2 servings

Prep time: 5 mins
Total time: 10 mins

Ingredients
3 eggs
2 1/2 oz cream cheese
1 tsp cinnamon
1 tbsp Swerve
1 tbsp butter

Directions
- Blend all ingredients together in a blender then let sit for 5 mins
- Divide batter for 2 pancakes and fry in melted butter
- Top with butter and sugar-free syrup

NOTE: You can double recipe and store remaining pancakes in the refrigerator and reheat

Nutritional Information per serving
235 calories
19.5 g fat
3.5 g carbohydrates
0.7 g fiber
12 g protein

Strawberry Smoothie

1 serving

Prep/total time: 5 mins

Ingredients
1 cup unsweetened coconut milk
1 tbsp vanilla
5 strawberries
2 tbsp heavy cream

Directions
- Blend all ingredients together until smooth

Nutritional Information per serving
165 calories
14 g fat
5.5 g carbohydrates
2 g fiber
0.5 g protein

Zucchini Bread

12 slices

Prep time: 10 mins
Total time: 1 hr

Ingredients
4 eggs
1-2 cups shredded zucchini, with moisture squeezed out
1/2 cup almond flour
1/4 cup coconut flour
8 tbsp coconut oil
1 tsp baking powder
1 tsp vanilla extract
dash of salt
dash of cinnamon

Directions
- Preheat oven to 350° F
- Mix all ingredients in a bowl
- Pour into greased loaf pan
- Bake 50 mins
- Let cool and slice

Nutritional Information per slice
152 calories
13.5 g fat
3.6 g carbohydrates
1.7 g fiber

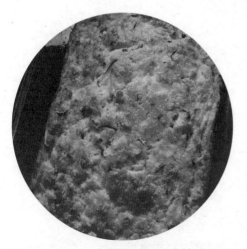

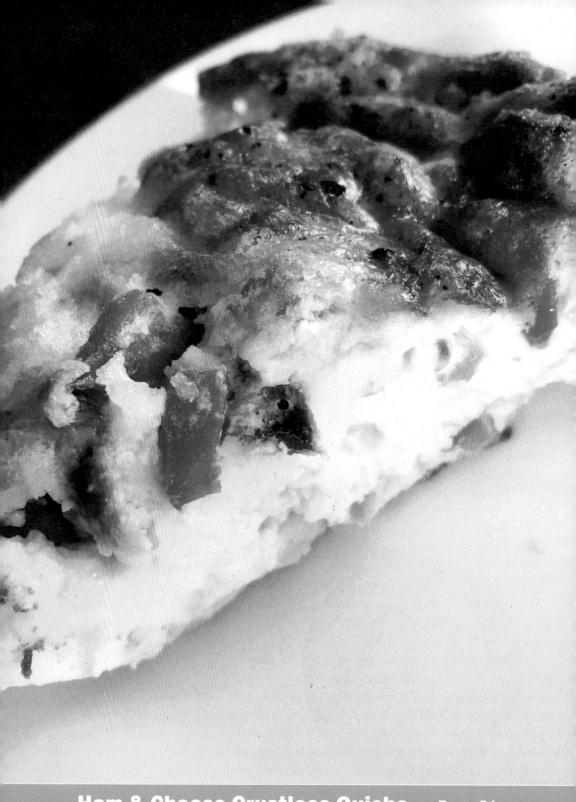

Ham & Cheese Crustless Quiche > Page 81

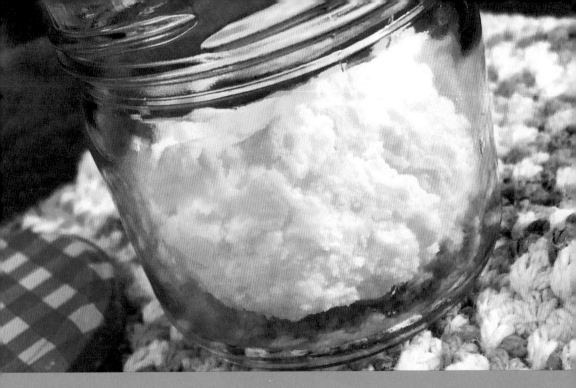

Mason Jar Homemade Butter > Page 116

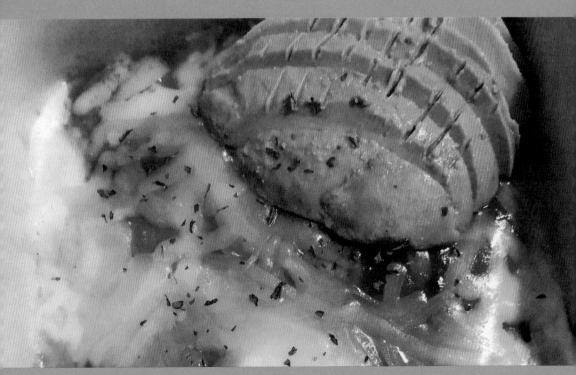

Pizza Eggs > Page 39

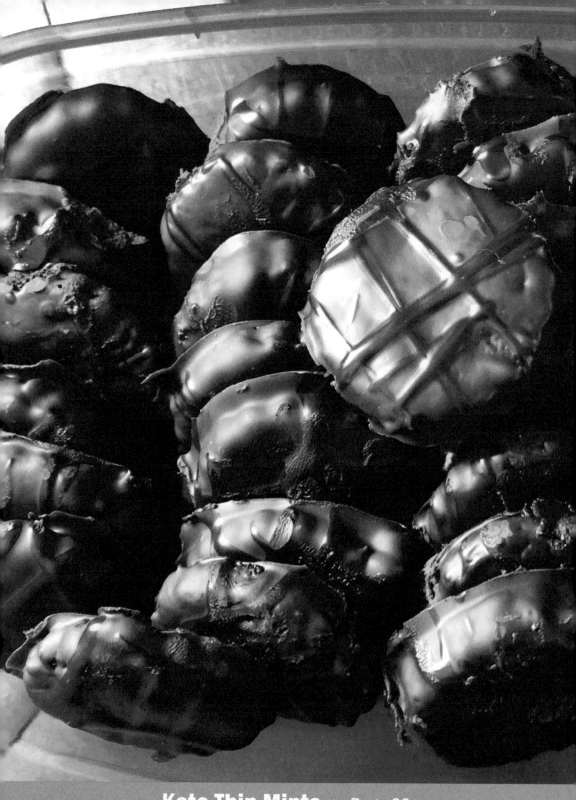

Keto Thin Mints > Page 66

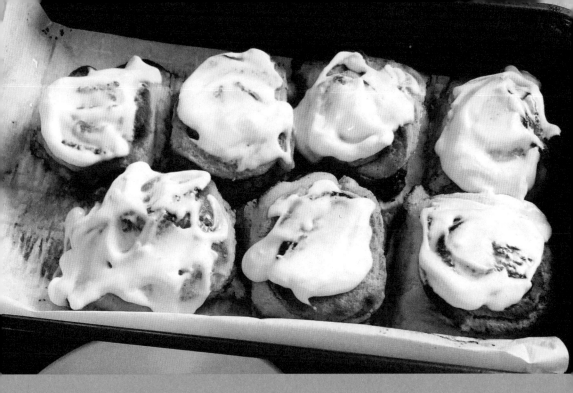

Cinnamon Rolls > Page 58

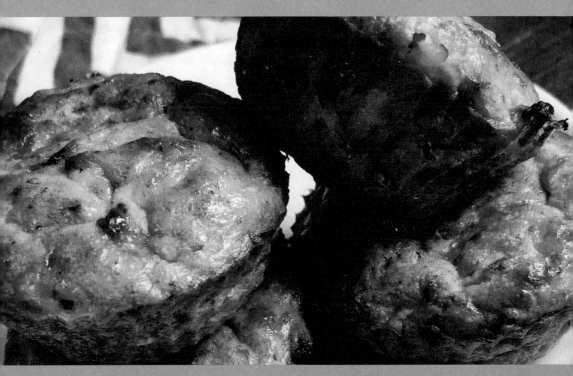

Tuna Melts > Page 108

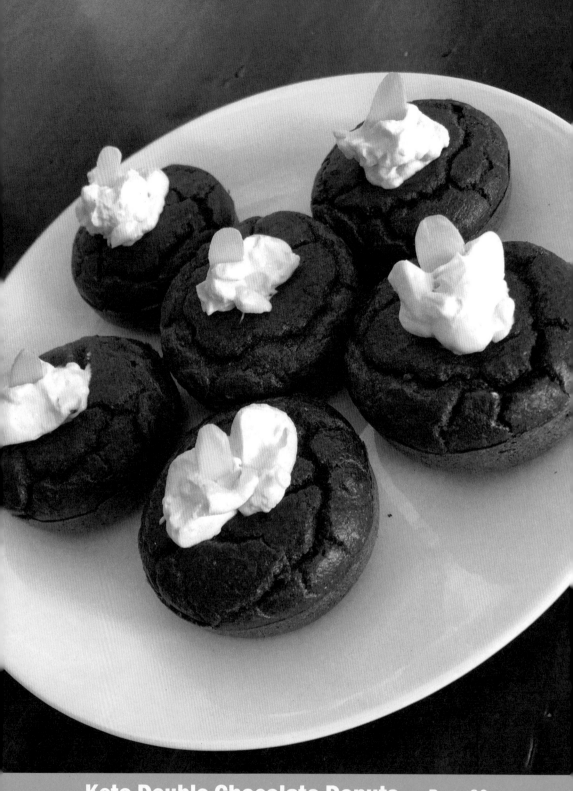

Keto Double Chocolate Donuts > Page 60

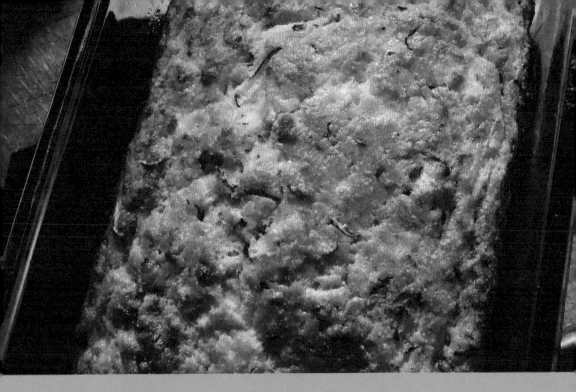

Zucchini Bread > Page 43

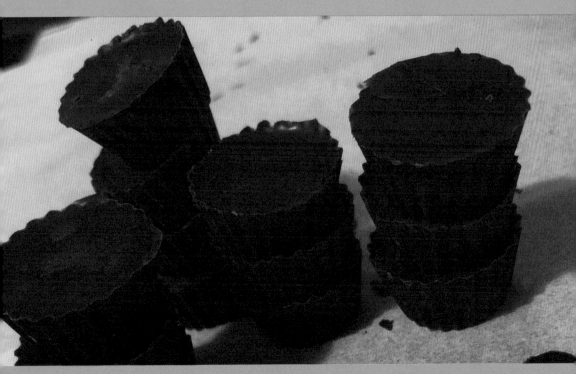

Peanut Butter Cup Fat Bombs > Page 64

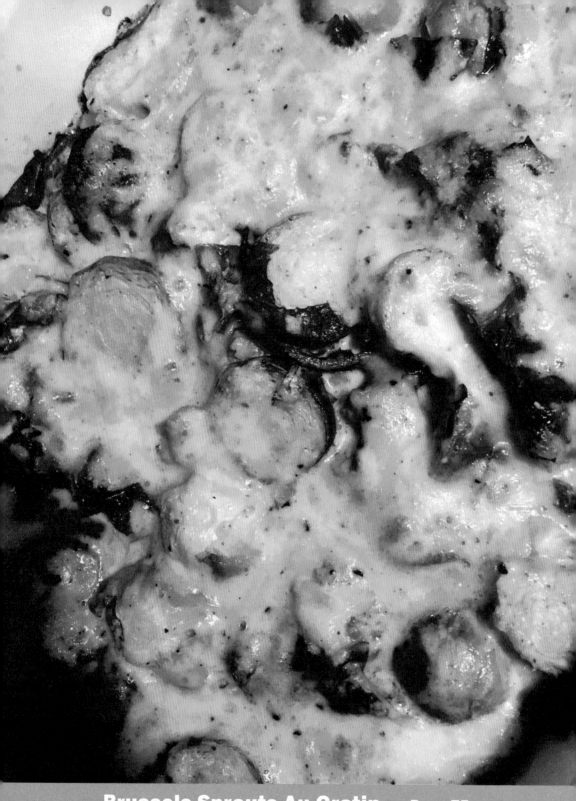

Brussels Sprouts Au Gratin > Page 75

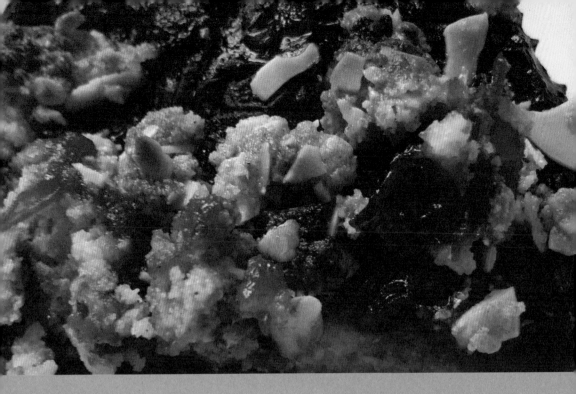

Cranberry Crumble > Page 59

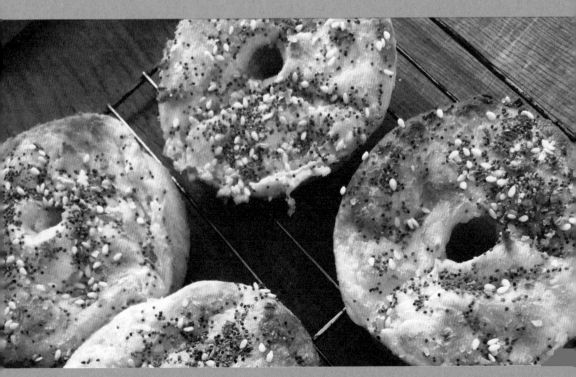

Bagels > Page 31

THE KETO SOLUTION

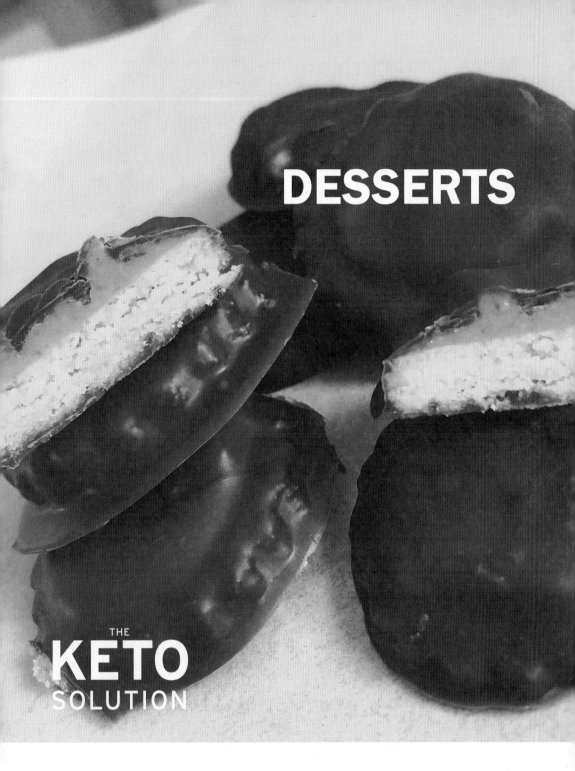

DESSERTS

Mock Apple Crisp

9 servings

Prep time: 5 mins
Total time: 50 mins

Ingredients
Filling
6 cups zucchini, peeled and sliced
3 tbsp lemon juice
2/3 cup Swerve sweetener
3/4 tsp ground cinnamon
1 tsp ground nutmeg

Topping
1/2 cup pecans, chopped
1/2 cup almond flour
1/4 cup coconut flour
1/4 cup Swerve
1 tsp cinnamon
1/4 cup butter

Directions
- Preheat oven to 350° F
- In a bowl, combine zucchini, lemon juice, sweetener, cinnamon, and nutmeg until well blended
- Pour mixture into a greased 9x9" baking dish
- To make the topping, combine pecans, almond flour, coconut flour, sweetener, and cinnamon in a bowl then cut in butter until crumbly
- Sprinkle over the zucchini mixture
- Bake for 45-50 mins or until zucchini is tender

Nutritional Information per serving
137 calories
13 g fat
6 g carbohydrates
3 g fiber
3 g protein

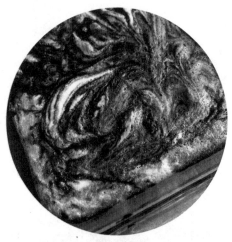

Blueberry Swirl Coffee Cake

9 servings

Prep time: 15 mins
Total time: 40 mins

Ingredients
Blueberry Swirl
3 tbsp granulated erythritol
1/4 tsp xanthan gum
2 tbsp water
1 tbsp lemon juice
1 cup blueberries, fresh or frozen

Cake Batter
1 1/2 cups superfine almond flour
1/3 cup granulated erythritol
1/4 tsp baking soda
1/8 tsp sea salt
2 tbsp butter or coconut oil, cut into large chunks
1/4 cup unsweetened almond milk
3 large eggs
1 tsp vanilla extract

Directions
- Preheat oven to 350° F
- Grease an 8x8" glass baking dish

Blueberry Swirl
-In a small saucepan, whisk together the erythritol and the xanthan; slowly add the water and the lemon juice while whisking
- Stir in the blueberries
- Bring mixture to a simmer over medium heat, then turn heat to low
- Simmer, stirring occasionally, until the mixture has the consistency of a thick blueberry syrup (about 5-10 mins); set aside

Cake Batter
- Place almond flour, granulated erythritol, baking soda, and sea salt in a food processor
- Pulse a few times to blend; add the butter or coconut oil and pulse again to incorporate
- In a separate bowl, whisk together the almond milk, eggs, and vanilla extract

- Slowly add the wet ingredients into dry mixture in the food processor, pulsing after each addition; pulse a few more times until batter is smooth
- Transfer batter to the prepared baking dish
- Spoon the blueberry syrup in strips on top of the batter
- Using a butter knife, swirl the batter to create the swirls
- Bake in the preheated oven for 25-28 mins; top should spring back when lightly touched
- Cut cake into 9 pieces
- Cover and refrigerate any leftovers

Nutritional Information per serving
88 calories
7 g fat
4 g carbohydrates
1 g fiber
3 g protein

Brownie Bombs

15 Servings

Prep time: 5 mins
Total time: 30 mins

Ingredients
1 8 oz block of cream cheese, softened
1/4 cup coconut oil
1/4 cup unsweetened cocoa powder
2/3 cup Krisda chocolate chips or other sugar-free chocolate

Directions
- In a large bowl combine cream cheese, coconut oil, and cocoa powder with hand mixer; fold in chocolate chips
- Use a small cookie scoop or tablespoon and place mixture onto a baking sheet lined with parchment paper
- Freeze for 20-30 mins, until set
- Store in freezer or refrigerator

Nutritional Information per serving
60 calories
5.9 g fat
4 g carbohydrates
2.3 g fiber
0.8 g protein

Chocolate Peanut Butter Squares

16 squares

Prep time: 20 mins
Total time: 20 mins

Squares
1 cup natural peanut butter
2/3 cup erythritol/Stevia sweetener, powdered
2 tbsp coconut flour
4 tbsp butter, melted

Topping
1/2 cup sugar free chocolate chips
1 tbsp butter
1 tbsp peanut butter

Directions
- Mix all the ingredients for the squares in a bowl with hand mixer until combined and creamy
- Spread into a lined 8x8" dish; freeze until set
- Add chocolate and 1 tbsp butter to a bowl and heat in 30-sec bursts; whisk until melted
- Spread over squares; freeze until set
- Heat tbsp peanut butter and drizzle it over the top
- Cut into 16 squares

Nutritional Information per serving
155 calories
12.5 g fat
9.5 g carbohydrates
4 g fiber
4.6 g Protein

Chocolate Truffles

20 chocolates, depending on mould size used

Prep time: 5 mins
Total time: 1 hr

Ingredients
4 tbsp butter
4 tbsp coconut oil
2 oz sugar-free chocolate chips, such as Lily's or Krisda
1/4 cup + 1 tbsp heavy cream
1/3 cup Swerve sweetener
2 tsp vanilla extract
nuts/shredded coconut for toppings (optional)

NOTE: An option is to replace vanilla extract with other flavours such as mint, orange, or cherry extracts

Directions
- Melt butter and coconut oil in microwave for 45 secs; whisk in chocolate
- Add heavy cream, sweetener, and vanilla; whisk until smooth
- Pour into silicone moulds; add toppings (if using)
- Freeze 1 hr until set; store in refrigerator

Nutritional Information per chocolate
62 calories
6.8 g fat
2.1 g carbohydrates
0.5 g fiber
0.1 g protein

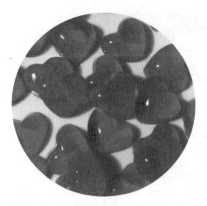

Keto Cinnamon Heart Gummies

1 serving (40 hearts)

Prep time: 5 mins
Total time: 30 mins (to set)

Ingredients
1 cup water
2 tbsp Swerve sweetener (optional)
8-10 drops cinnamon oil
3 tbsp gelatin powder

Directions
- Mix the first three ingredients together in a pot stovetop over medium heat until very warm
- Gradually mix in gelatin powder until fully dissolved
- Transfer to silicone moulds and refrigerate 30 mins until set

Nutritional Information per serving
115 calories
4 g fat
23 g carbohydrates
16 g fiber
1.7 g protein

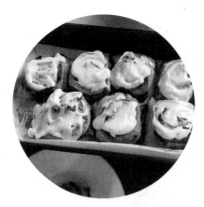

Cinnamon Rolls

10 servings

Prep time: 15 mins
Total time: 30 mins

Ingredients
Dough
2 cups shredded mozzarella cheese
3 oz cream cheese
2 eggs
1 tsp vanilla
3/4 cup coconut flour
1/2 tsp xanthan gum
1/2 tsp salt
1 tbsp baking powder
1/4 cup Swerve sweetener

Cinnamon "sugar" filling
1/2 cup butter, melted
2 tsp ground cinnamon

Cream cheese frosting
3 tbsp heavy cream
3 oz cream cheese
1 tbsp Swerve
1/2 tsp vanilla extract
1/4 tsp almond extract

Directions
- Preheat oven to 400° F
- Combine the cream cheese and shredded cheese in a bowl and heat for 2 mins; mix
- Add remaining dough ingredients and mix thoroughly
- Place dough between two sheets of parchment paper and roll out to roughly 16x8"
- Cut into 10 strips
- Combine the ingredients for the "sugar" mix and mix well; spread half the mixture onto strips
- Roll strips into cinnamon rolls; you can use a rubber spatula to assist
- Sprinkle remaining "sugar" mix on top of the cinnamon rolls
- Bake 15-18 mins
- While cinnamon rolls are baking you can make your cream cheese frosting by placing all the ingredients in a blender and mixing
- Spread over top when cinnamon rolls are done and cooled a little

Nutritional Information per serving
270 calories
23 g fat
6.6 g carbohydrates
3.2 g fiber
9.5 g protein

Cranberry Crumble

16 servings

Prep time: 30 mins
Total time: 1 hr

Ingredients
Shortbread crust
6 tbsp butter, melted
2 cups almond flour
1/2 cup erythritol granulated
sweetener
1/2 tsp almond extract

Cranberry filling
2 cups fresh or frozen cranberries
1/2 cup erythritol granulated
sweetener
1/4 cup water
1/4 tsp xanthan gum

Streusel topping
1/3 crust mix (from above)
1/2 tsp ground cinnamon
1/4 cup chopped pecans/almonds

Directions
Crust
- Combine all of the crust ingredients in a medium-sized bowl and mix well with a fork
- Remove approximately 1/3 of the crust mix and set aside for the streusel topping
- Press the remaining 2/3 of the crust mix into an 8x8" baking pan, preferably lined with parchment or foil for easier removal after baking
- Bake in a 350° F preheated oven for 5 mins
- Remove and set aside

Cranberry filling
- In a small saucepan, combine cranberries, sweetener, water, and xanthan gum and stir well
- Bring to a boil; simmer on low heat for 10 mins
- Stir and pop all of the cranberries that remained whole after cooking
- Remove from heat and cool for about five mins, or until no longer steaming
- Spread the cranberry filling evenly over the partially baked shortbread crust

Streusel topping
- Add cinnamon and chopped pecans to the 1/3 crust mix you set aside earlier
- Work mixture with your fingers until clusters are formed
- Sprinkle the streusel evenly over the cranberry layer
- Bake bars at 350° F for 30 mins
- Remove from oven and cool before slicing

Nutritional Information per serving
136 calories
11 g fat
6 g carbohydrates
3 g fiber
4 g protein

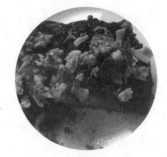

Crock Pot Fudge

20 pieces

Prep time: 5 mins
Total time: 3 hrs

Ingredients
2 1/2 cups sugar-free chocolate
1/3 cup coconut milk
1 tsp vanilla
2 tbsp sweetener

Directions
- Stir ingredients into a crock pot
- Cover and cook on low for 2 hrs
- Uncover, turn off, and let sit for 30-50 mins; do not stir
- After 30-50 mins stir well until smooth
- Line a quart casserole dish with parchment paper and spread in mixture
- Chill until firm

Nutritional Information per piece
63 calories
6.6 g fat
3.8 g carbohydrates
1.6 g fiber
1.3 g protein

Keto Double Chocolate Donuts

6 donuts

Prep time: 10 mins
Total time: 30 mins

Ingredients
1/4 cup coconut flour
1/4 cup cocoa powder
1/8 tsp sea salt
1/2 tsp baking soda
3 eggs
1/4 cup coconut oil, melted
1/3 cup sugar-free maple syrup
(such as Walden Farms)
1 tbsp vanilla extract

Chocolate glaze for topping
2 oz sugar-free chocolate
2 tbsp coconut oil, melted

Directions
- Preheat oven to 350° F
- In a medium bowl whisk together coconut flour, cocoa powder, sea salt, and baking soda
- Add eggs, coconut oil, syrup, and vanilla; whisk until batter forms
- Transfer to silicone donut mould and bake 18-20 mins until dough has risen and it is firm to the touch

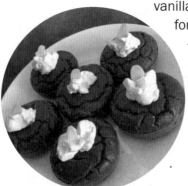

- Cool 15 mins; transfer to wire rack to cool completely
- Melt glaze ingredients together and dip donuts

Nutritional Information per donut
157 calories
12.9 g fat
5.2 g carbohydrates
3 g fiber
4.5 g protein

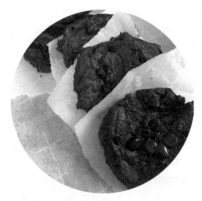

Flourless Chocolate Chip Cookies

18 cookies

Prep time: 10 mins
Total time: 22 mins

Ingredients
1 cup almond butter
2/3 cup confectioners Swerve
2 tbsp cocoa powder, unsweetened
2 tbsp peanut butter powder
2 eggs
1 tbsp salted butter, melted
2 tbsp water
1 1/2 tsp vanilla extract
1 tsp baking soda
1/4 cup sugar-free chocolate chips (Krisda or Lily's)

Directions
- Preheat oven to 350° F
- Line a baking sheet with a silicone baking mat or parchment paper
- In a mixing bowl, combine almond butter, erythritol, cocoa powder, peanut butter powder, eggs, butter, water, vanilla extract, and baking soda
- Using an electric hand mixer, mix until all ingredients are well combined, creating a very thick dough.
- Fold in chocolate chips
- Form the dough into 1 1/2-2" balls
- Place the cookie dough on the prepared baking sheet
- Bake for 8-10 mins (begin checking on them at 8 mins)
- Remove the baking sheet from the oven and place on a cooling rack

Nutritional Information per cookie
115 calories
10 g fat
3.8 g carbohydrates
2.5 g fiber
4 g protein

French Toast Donuts

6 donuts

Prep time: 5 mins
Total time: 25 mins

Ingredients
1/2 cup butter, melted
1/4 cup heavy cream
1/4 cup swerve sweetener
4 eggs
1 tbsp vanilla
1/4 cup coconut flour
1 tbsp baking powder

Directions
- Preheat oven to 350° F
- Blend butter, cream and sweetener
- Add eggs and vanilla; blend well
- Add baking powder and coconut flour, blend well
- Spoon into silicone mould or greased donut pan
- Bake 15-20 mins
- Mix 2 tbsp sweetener and 1 tsp cinnamon together and dip donuts (optional)

Nutritional Information per donut
237 calories
22 g fat
2.9 g carbohydrates
1.7 g fiber
5.2 g protein

Keto Gummy Bears

1 serving (18-20 bears)

Prep time: 5 mins
Total time: 25 mins (to set)

Ingredients
1 box sugar-free Jell-O
.25 oz (7 g) gelatin powder
1/2 cup hot water

Directions
- Mix all ingredients until Jell-O and gelatin are fully dissolved
- Transfer to silicone moulds and refrigerate 25-30 mins until set

Nutritional Information per serving
33 calories
0 g fat
0 g carbohydrates
0 g fiber
7.3 g protein

Keto Homemade Frosties

4 servings

Prep time: 5 mins
Total time: 35 mins

Ingredients
1 1/2 cups heavy whipping cream
2 tbsp cocoa powder
3 tbsp Swerve sweetener
1 tsp vanilla extract
pinch of sea salt

Directions

- Blend all ingredients together until stiff peaks form
- Scoop into a Ziploc bag and freeze 30 mins
- Cut off tip of Ziploc bag and pipe into bowls

Nutritional Information per serving
305 calories
30 g fat
0.5 g carbohydrates
0.5 g fiber
2.1 g protein

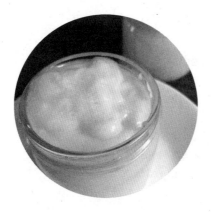

Lemon Curd
4 servings

Prep time: 5 mins
Total time: 5 mins

Ingredients
1/2 cup butter
1/2 cup Swerve sweetener
1/2 cup fresh lemon juice
1/4 cup lemon zest
6 egg yolks

Directions
- Melt butter in a pot on low heat
- Remove from heat and whisk in lemon zest, lemon juice, and sweetener until dissolved
- Whisk in yolks and return to heat; whisk continually until curd forms, about 5-10 mins
- Remove from heat and pour into small bowls; let cool to room temperature then cover and refrigerate for up to 1 month

Nutritional Information per serving
321 calories
29 g fat
12 g carbohydrates
0 g fiber
4.3 g protein

Keto Chocolate Mug Cake
1 serving

Prep/Total time: 5 mins

Ingredients
2 tbsp butter, melted
1 egg
2 tbsp cocoa powder
2 tbsp swerve sweetener
1 tbsp heavy whipping cream
1 tsp vanilla extract

Directions
- Mix together the egg and melted butter
- Add remaining ingredients and whisk together
- Microwave 90 secs

Nutritional Information per serving
265 calories
23 g fat
8.1 g carbohydrates
4.5 g fiber
9.3 g protein

No-bake Cookie Dough Bars

10 servings

Prep time: 10 mins
Total time: 20 mins

Ingredients
Bars
3/4 cup almond flour
2 tbsp coconut flour
1/3 cup Krisda chocolate chips
2 tbsp Walden Farms maple syrup
1/2 cup peanut butter, or any creamy nut butter

Topping
3 oz Krisda chocolate chips
2 tbsp peanut butter
1 tsp vanilla extract

Directions
- In a medium bowl add maple syrup and peanut butter; microwave 30 secs to warm up and mix together
- Add almond flour, coconut flour, and chocolate chips
- Stir until fully combined and dough forms
- Transfer to a lined loaf pan, press dough in, and freeze while melting topping
- In a bowl heat topping ingredients in 30-sec intervals until fully melted; mix
- Layer chocolate on top of cookie dough and freeze 10-15 mins until set
- Store in refrigerator

Nutritional Information per serving
234 calories
18 g fat
12.6 g carbohydrates
3.6 g fiber
6.8 g protein

Peanut Butter Cup Fat Bombs

12 servings

Prep time: 5 mins
Total time: 5 mins

Ingredients
2 tbsp coconut oil
2 tbsp butter
4 tbsp natural peanut butter
3 tbsp cocoa powder
3 packets Stevia
1 tsp vanilla extract

Directions
- Mix all ingredients together and heat in a microwave-safe dish for 30 secs and stir; if not fully dissolved return to microwave another 20-30 secs
- Pour into silicone moulds and freeze 30 mins
- Store in refrigerator or freezer in airtight container

Nutritional Information per serving
75 calories
7.1 g fat
1.8 g carbohydrates
0.8 g fiber
1.5 g protein

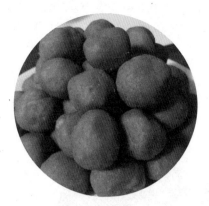

No-bake Peanut Butter Ball Bites
40 servings

Prep Time: 2 mins
Total Time: 30 mins

Ingredients
2 cups smooth natural peanut butter
1/2 cup sticky sweetener, such as
Walden Farms maple syrup or Mrs.
Butterworth's No Sugar Added syrup
3/4 cup coconut flour

Directions
- Line a baking tray or plate with
  parchment paper
- In a bowl mix all the ingredients
  together and combine well; if batter
  is too thick add a little almond milk
- Using your hands form the dough
  into small balls and place on lined
  tray
- Refrigerate 30 mins or until firm

Nutritional Information per serving
57 calories
4 g fat
3 g carbohydrates
1.5 g fiber
2 g protein

Pecan Pie
12 servings

Prep time: 5 mins
Total time: 20 mins

Ingredients
Crust
1 cup coconut flour
1/2 cup butter, melted
2 cups pecans

Glaze
1/2 cup butter
1/4 cup Swerve sweetener
1 tbsp vanilla extract

Directions
- Preheat oven to 350° F
- For the crust mix melted butter and
  coconut flour together and press
  into pie plate; top with pecans
- For the glaze, over medium heat
  melt butter, add sweetener and boil
  until browned, about 5 mins
- Pour over the pecans
- Bake 15 mins
- Let cool and serve with whipped
  cream

Nutritional Information per serving
304 calories
29.8 g fat
12 g carbohydrates
5 g fiber
3.2 g protein

Sweet Spiced Walnuts

7 Cups

Prep time: 10 mins
Total time: 30 mins

Ingredients
5 cups walnuts, halves or pieces
1 egg white
1 cup sweetener
1 tsp ground cinnamon
1/4 tsp ground nutmeg
1/4 tsp ground allspice
1/4 salt

Directions
- Preheat oven to 325° F
- Grease or line a 9x13" (or larger) baking pan
- In a bowl combine egg white and 1 tsp water
- Add nuts; toss to coat
- In a separate bowl combine sweetener, spices, and salt
- Sprinkle mixture over the nuts and toss to coat fully
- Spread the nuts onto the pan and bake for 20 mins
- Spread onto a piece of parchment paper and let cool
- Break into pieces if using halves and store in an airtight container

Nutritional Information per 2 tbsp
84 calories
7 g fat
5 g carbohydrates
1 g fiber
2 g protein

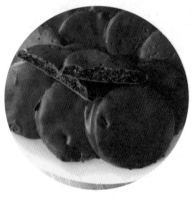

Keto Thin Mints

20 cookies

Prep time: 30 mins
Total time: 1 hr

Ingredients
Cookies
1 3/4 cups almond flour
1/3 cup cocoa powder
1/3 cup Swerve
1 egg, beaten
1 tsp baking powder
1/2 tsp salt
2 tbsp butter, melted
1/2 tsp vanilla extract

Coating
1 tbsp coconut oil
7 oz sugar-free chocolate
1 tsp peppermint extract

Directions
- Preheat the oven to 300° F; line two baking sheets with parchment paper
- In large bowl combine almond flour, cocoa powder, sweetener, baking powder, and salt
- Add in egg, butter, and vanilla and stir well until dough forms
- Roll out dough between two pieces of parchment paper to no more than 1/4" thick; lift off top paper
- Using a 2"-diameter cookie cutter, cut out circles of dough and lift gently; place cookies on prepared baking sheet
- Reroll extra dough and cut out until there is too little to use
- Bake cookies until firm to the touch, 20 mins or so, depending on how thinly you rolled your dough; remove and let cool
- For the chocolate coating, melt chocolate and coconut oil together, either in the microwave or on stovetop; stir until smooth; remove from heat and add peppermint extract
- Dip cookies into the chocolate mixture using two forks, letting the excess chocolate drip off, and place on lined baking sheet
- Refrigerate until fully set

Nutritional Information per 2 cookies
116 calories
10 g fat
6.99 g carbohydrates
4.81 g fiber
3.08 g protein

THE KETO SOLUTION

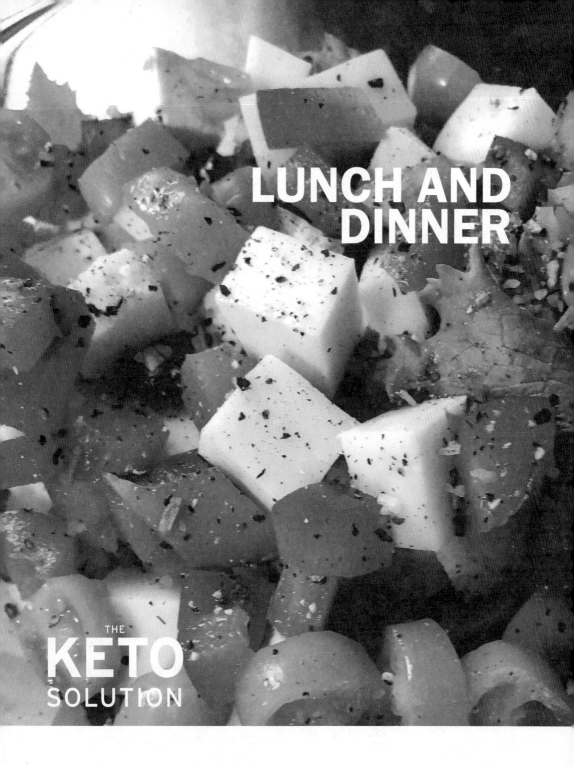

LUNCH AND DINNER

THE
KETO
SOLUTION

Avocado Chicken Curry

4 servings

Prep time: 10 mins
Total time: 20 mins

Ingredients
1 LB boneless skinless chicken thighs
2 avocados
2 cups almond or coconut milk
1 tbsp curry powder
1 tbsp garlic powder
1/2 tsp salt
1/2 tsp pepper
1 cup broccoli
1 cup cauliflower
1 cup green pepper

Directions
- Blend avocado, milk, and spices in blender
- Cook chopped chicken in butter
- Add veggies and soften for 5 min
- Add curry; mix
- Simmer 5 mins

Nutritional Information per serving
294 calories
16.4 g fat
13.9 g carbohydrates
7.7 g fiber
25.6 g protein

Bacon Cheeseburger Casserole

12 servings

Prep time: 20 mins
Total time: 55 mins

Ingredients
2 LB ground beef
2 cloves garlic, minced
1 tsp onion powder
1 lb bacon, cooked and chopped
8 eggs
1 can (6 OZ) tomatoes
1 cup heavy cream
1/2 tsp salt
1 tsp pepper
12 oz shredded cheddar cheese, divided

Directions
- Preheat oven to 350° F
- Brown the ground beef with garlic and onion powder
- Drain, then spread beef on the bottom of a 9x13" casserole dish
- Stir bacon pieces into ground beef
- In a medium bowl whisk together eggs, tomato paste, heavy cream, salt, and pepper until well combined
- Stir 8 oz of shredded cheese into egg mixture
- Pour egg mixture over ground beef and bacon
- Top with remaining shredded cheese

- Bake at 350° F for 30-35 mins or until golden on the top

Nutritional Information per serving
587 calories
49 g fat
4 g carbohydrates
0.2 g fiber
29 g protein

Bacon Goat Cheese Avocado Salad
4 servings

Prep time: 10 mins
Total time: 15 mins

Ingredients
Salad
8 oz goat cheese
3 slices bacon
2 avocados
1/4 cup chopped walnuts
4 cups arugula lettuce

Dressing
1/2 lemon, juiced
2 tbsp mayo
2 tbsp olive oil
2 tbsp heaving whipping cream

Directions
- Preheat oven to 400° F; place parchment paper on a baking sheet
- Cut the goat cheese into round ½-1-inch slices and place on the baking sheet; bake on upper rack until golden
- Fry the bacon in a pan until crispy
- Cut the avocado into pieces and place on top of the arugula lettuce
- Add fried bacon and goat cheese and sprinkle with walnuts
- Mix all dressing ingredients together with a stick blender
- Add salt and pepper to taste

Nutritional Information per serving
520 calories
47 g fat
10 g carbohydrates
6 g fiber
16 g protein

Keto Rolls

6 rolls

Prep time: 5 mins
Total time: 1 hr

Ingredients
1 1/4 cups almond flour
5 tbsp psyllium husk powder
2 tsp baking powder
1 tsp salt
2 tsp apple cider vinegar
1 cup boiling water
3 egg whites
1/4 tsp yeast for bread flavour
(optional)

Directions
- Preheat oven to 350° F
- Add all dry ingredients together
  and mix
- Add boiling water, egg, and vinegar
- Mix 30 secs; do not overmix
- Divide into rolls, buns, or flatbread
- Bake 50 mins

Nutritional Information per roll
170 calories
11 g fat
9.7 g carbohydrates
9 g fiber
7 g protein

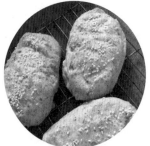

Big Mac in a Bowl

2 servings

Prep time: 15 mins
Total time: 25 mins

Ingredients
16 oz ground beef
6 cups romaine lettuce
1/4 cup red onion, diced
2 dill pickle spears, chopped
1/4 cup shredded cheddar cheese
4 tbsp Walden Farms Thousand
Island dressing
salt and pepper, to taste

Directions
- Brown ground beef until cooked
  through; drain
- Chop romaine lettuce
- Chop red onion and pickles; set
  aside
- Pour Thousand Island dressing
  onto lettuce as desired; mix until
  evenly coated
- Add ground beef and chopped
  vegetables to the lettuce and mix
  until coated
- Add salt and pepper

Nutritional Information per serving
480 calories
29 g fat
5 g carbohydrates
2 g fiber
51 g protein

"Bread" Sticks

2 servings

Prep time: 5 mins
Total time: 25 mins

Ingredients
1 cup shredded mozzarella
1/4 cup Parmesan cheese
1 egg
1 slice of bacon, precooked and cut up
1 tsp garlic powder, or to taste
jalapenos (optional)

Directions
- Preheat oven to 350° F
- Mix all ingredients in a bowl, except jalapenos and bacon
- Spread out onto parchment paper; top with jalapenos and bacon
- Bake for 20 mins
  -Serve with low-sugar marinara sauce

Nutritional Information per serving
338 calories
24 g fat
2.9 g carbohydrates
0 g fiber
26 g protein

Broccoli Cheddar Soup

4 servings

Prep time: 10 mins
Total time: 40 mins

Ingredients
4 cups broccoli florets, chopped
3 cups sharp cheddar cheese, shredded
2 pieces bacon (optional)
1/4 medium onion, diced
5 cloves fresh garlic, pressed
2 celery stalks, diced
2 cups bone broth
2 cups heavy whipping cream
1/4 tsp pink Himalayan salt
1/2 tsp black peppercorns

Directions
- Cook bacon strips in a large saucepan on medium heat for 2-3 mins per side until crispy; remove and set aside for garnish
- Place onion, celery, and garlic into the pot and cook for about 10 mins; stir occasionally, cooking until onions start to become translucent
- Season the vegetables with the pink Himalayan salt and ground black pepper
- Add in broccoli and bone broth, and stir for about 1 min

...more

continued...

- Add in whipping cream and simmer for an additional 9 mins on medium heat
- Slowly start adding in the shredded cheddar cheese after the broccoli has been cooking for 10 mins; add in about 1 cup at a time, and stir for about 1 min in between
- Continue to simmer for about 10 mins
- When ready to serve, serve the soup hot, and with the optional garnish of more shredded cheddar cheese and the crumbled bacon from earlier

Nutritional Information per serving
520 calories
45 g fat
11 g carbohydrates
3 g fiber
26 g protein

Broccoli Salad
6 servings

Prep time: 5 mins
Total time: 10 mins

Ingredients
24 oz fresh broccoli
1 cup mayo
1/4 cup Swerve sweetener
1 tbsp apple cider vinegar
1/2 cup bacon, cooked and crumbled
1/4 cup red onion
1/4 cup crushed nuts of choice

Directions
- Cut up broccoli and onion; add nuts and bacon
- In a bowl mix mayo, sweetener, and vinegar until combined; add to broccoli and onion
- Stir to coat; add fresh pepper

Nutritional Information per serving
455 calories
43 g fat
16 g carbohydrates
3 g fiber
7.8 g protein

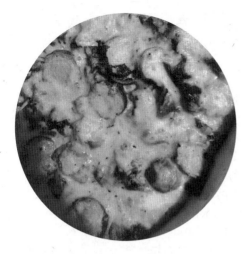

bacon
- Coat cooked Brussels sprouts with mixture
- Top with crumbled bacon
- Bake 30 mins

Nutritional Information per serving
400 calories
15 g fat
8 g carbohydrates
2.1 g fiber
11.4 g protein

Brussels Sprouts Au Gratin
Makes 8 servings

Prep time: 15 mins
Total time: 45 mins

1 lb Brussels sprouts
2 tbsp avocado oil or bacon fat
1/2 tsp salt
1/2 tsp pepper
1 egg
1/2 cup whipping cream
1/2 tsp red pepper flakes
1 tsp onion powder
1 tsp garlic powder
2 cups cheese
4 slices bacon, crumbled

Directions
- Preheat oven to 350° F
- Halve Brussels sprouts
- Coat in oil, salt and pepper
- Bake 15 min
- Mix all other ingredients except

Buffalo Chicken and Broccoli Bowls
4 servings

Prep time: 10 mins
Total time: 30 mins

Ingredients
Riced Cauliflower
1 head cauliflower
1 tbsp olive oil
salt and pepper

Buffalo Chicken and Broccoli
1 lb boneless, skinless chicken thighs, cut into bite-sized pieces
2 large heads of broccoli, cut into small florets
1 tbsp olive oil
1/4 cup hot sauce
2 tbsp butter
salt and pepper

...more

continued...

Directions
Riced cauliflower
- Cut into small florets
- Working in small batches, place florets into a food processor; pulse until cauliflower resembles grains of rice, about 20 pulses; do not over-process
- Heat olive oil in a pan over medium heat; add cauliflower and season with salt and pepper
- Sauté until tender for 5-8 mins

Buffalo chicken and broccoli
- Heat a skillet that has a lid over medium heat; add oil, if using, and when hot add chicken
- Season with a small amount of salt
- Allow to cool on one side until browned, then turn and brown the other side; cook until no longer pink, about 4-5 min per side
- When chicken is cooked, add broccoli to the pan and cover
- Allow to steam until tender for 5-10 mins, stirring a few times; broccoli is done wen easily pierced and still bright green
- Meanwhile, prepare buffalo sauce; melt 2 tbsp butter with the hot sauce and whisk to combine
- Pour sauce over the chicken and broccoli; toss to coat
- Serve over riced cauliflower

Nutritional Information per serving
315 calories
17.8 g fat
15.2 g carbohydrates
6.5 g fiber
28 g protein

Butter Chicken
6 servings

Prep time: 30 mins
Total time: 30 mins

Ingredients
1/2 cup chopped onion
1/4 cup butter
1 1/2 tsp garam masala spice
1 tsp chili powder
1 tsp cumin
1 tsp ginger powder
1 tsp minced garlic
1 tbsp lemon juice
4 cups cooked chicken
1 cup tomato sauce
1 cup 18% cream
3/4 cup plain full-fat yogurt
6 cups cauliflower rice

Directions
- Sauté onions in butter until soft; add remaining ingredients and cook for 1-2 mins
- Add tomato sauce, cream, and yogurt
- Mix in 4 cups cooked chicken and serve over cauliflower rice or other cooked vegetables

Nutritional Information per serving:
370 calories
13 g carbohydrates
20 g protein
3 g fiber
27.5 g fat

Smoky Cheese Ball
3 1/2 cups

Prep time: 30 mins
Total time: 4 hrs (chill time)

Ingredients
16 oz cream cheese
2 cups finely shredded cheese
(cheddar, Swiss, or gouda)
1/2 cup butter
2 tbsp cream
2 tsp steak sauce (low/sugar-free)
1 cup nuts, finely chopped

Directions
- Let cream cheese, shredded
  cheese, and butter stand at room
  temperature for 30 mins
- Add cream and steak sauce; beat
  until fluffy
- Cover and chill for up to 4 hrs
- Shape into a ball and roll in
  chopped nuts
- Serve with keto rolls or veggies

NOTE: If you prefer flavour other than
smoke, you can omit the steak sauce
and add other flavours such as garlic
and onion or dill, as examples.

Nutritional Information (per 1 tbsp)
73 calories
7 g fat
1 g carbohydrates
0 g fiber
2 g protein

Cheese Ball
Makes approximately 16 servings

Prep time: 30 mins
Total time: 2 hrs (chill time)

Ingredients
2 8-OZ packages full-fat cream
cheese, softened
3 cups grated cheddar cheese
2 tbsp onion/chive dip spice
1 tbsp lemon juice
1/4 tsp white pepper
1/8 tsp sea salt (may add more to
taste)
1/2 cup crushed pecans

Directions
- Mix cheeses, spice, lemon juice,
  salt, and pepper
- Shape into a ball and roll in
  chopped nuts
- Serve with keto rolls or veggies

Nutritional Information per serving
(approximately 5 tbsp):
194 calories
2 g carbohydrates
14 g fat
0.2 g fiber
4 g protein

Cheese Biscuit\
Hamburger Rolls
16 servings

Prep time: 15 mins
Total time: 30 mins

Ingredients
3 cups almond flour
1 cup sour cream
2 tbsp baking powder
4 oz melted butter
2 cups shredded cheese
4 eggs

Directions
- Preheat oven to 400° F
- Mix all ingredients
- Chill 15 mins
- Shape into approximately 16 biscuits/buns
- Bake 15 mins

Nutritional Information per biscuit/roll
179 calories
17 g fat
1.8 g carbohydrates
0.6 g fiber
6.7 g protein

Cloud Bread
10 pieces

Prep time: 10 mins
Total time: 40 mins

Ingredients
4 eggs, room temperature
2 oz cream cheese, softened
1/4 tsp cream of tartar
1/4 tsp salt

Directions
- Preheat oven to 300° F and line two baking sheets with parchment paper
- Carefully separate egg whites from yolks, with whites in one bowl and yolks in another
- In the bowl of egg yolks, add cream cheese; mix together with a hand mixer until well combined
- In the bowl of egg whites, add cream of tartar and salt; using hand mixer, mix together at high speed until stiff peaks form
- Pouring slowly, carefully fold in yolk mixture to egg whites until there are no white streaks
- Spoon mixture onto prepared baking sheet about 1/2 to 3/4 inches tall and about 5 inches apart
- Bake in oven on middle rack for 30 mins, until tops are lightly golden
- Allow to cool as they form up while cooling

NOTE: Spices such as garlic powder or Italian season can also be added to the batter.

Nutritional Information per serving
50 calories
3.7 g fat
0.5 g carbohydrates
0 g fiber
2.9 g protein

Colourful Cabbage Salad

6 servings

Prep time: 10 mins
Total time: 15 mins

Ingredients
4 cups green cabbage, shredded
3 cups red cabbage, shredded
1/4 cup red bell pepper, chopped
1/2 cup green onion, thinly sliced
1/2 cup apple cider vinegar
4 tbsp Swerve sweetener
2 tsp pepper

Directions
- Toss green and red cabbage, green onion, and bell pepper in a large bowl
- Mix vinegar, sweetener, and pepper in a separate bowl
- Add dressing to cabbage mixture and mix well
- Refrigerate before serving

Nutritional Information per serving
70 calories
1 g fat
16 g carbohydrates
5 g fiber
3 g protein

Crack Slaw

4 servings

Prep time: 5 mins
Total time: 25 mins

Ingredients
2 tbsp sesame oil
3 cloves garlic, minced
1/2 cup onion, diced
5 green onions (optional)
1 lb ground beef
1/2 tsp ground ginger
1 tbsp sriracha or chili sauce
14 oz bag coleslaw
3 tbsp soy sauce
1 tbsp vinegar
sweetener to taste
sea salt and pepper to taste

Directions
- Heat sesame oil in a large skillet over medium heat
- Add garlic and onions and sauté until the onions are translucent and the garlic is fragrant
- Add ground beef, ginger, salt, pepper, and sriracha
- Sauté until meat is cooked through
- Add coleslaw mix, soy sauce, and vinegar
- Sauté until coleslaw is tender

Nutritional Information per serving
312 calories
19 g fat
7 g carbohydrates
3 g fiber
26 g protein

Creamy Bacon Skillet

4 servings

Prep time: 10 mins
Total time: 20 mins

Ingredients
4 eggs
1 tbsp bacon fat (from previously cooked bacon)
1/2 head of cabbage, grated
4 mushrooms, chopped
1 tbsp minced garlic
1 small yellow onion, chopped
2 tbsp ranch dressing OR sour cream
1/4 block cream cheese
1/2 cup grated Parmesan
1/2 cup shredded mozzarella cheese
4 strips of bacon, cooked and chopped
1/4 cup heavy cream
salt and pepper to taste

Directions
- In a pan cook bacon (save fat); let cool and chop
- In a separate pan, scramble eggs; remove and set aside
- Add bacon fat to the pan on medium/heat; add grated cabbage and chopped mushrooms
- Add salt, pepper, minced garlic, and chopped onion; stir; cover and simmer until soft
- Add ranch dressing or sour cream, cream cheese, Parmesan, shredded cheese, bacon, heavy cream, and eggs
- Stir well; cover and simmer until cheese is melted

Nutritional Information per serving
434 calories
32 g fat
14 g carbohydrates
4.2 g fiber
23.6 g protein

Crusted Chicken Strips

4 servings

Prep time: 5 mins
Total time: 30 mins

Ingredients
1½ lb chicken, boneless and skinless
2 cups crushed pork rinds
1/2 cup grated Parmesan cheese
1 tsp garlic powder
1 tsp onion powder
1 tsp cumin
1/4 tsp salt
1/2 tsp pepper
1 egg

Directions
- Preheat oven to 350° F
- Cut chicken into strips (whole breasts, if desired)
- Combine all dry ingredients in a bowl and mix
- In a separate bowl whisk the egg
- Dip chicken into egg and roll in crust mixture
- Bake on a lined baking sheet for 25-30 mins until cooked through

Nutritional Information per serving
500 calories
27 g fat
2.8 g carbohydrates
0 g fiber
60 g protein

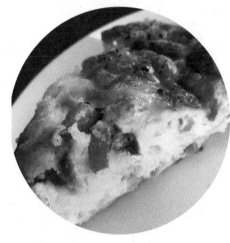

Ham and Cheese Crustless Quiche

8 servings

Prep timé: 10 mins
Total time: 45 mins

Ingredients
8 oz shredded cheddar cheese
6 eggs
1 cup heavy cream
8 oz ham, cubed
1/2 cup onion, diced
2 cups broccoli florets
1 tbsp butter
salt and pepper to taste

Directions
- Preheat oven to 375° F
- In a skillet over medium high heat, melt butter and add onions and ham
- Sauté for 5-7 mins until onions are translucent
- Place broccoli in a microwave-safe bowl and add 2 tbsp water
- Microwave for 2-3 mins until broccoli is lightly steamed and tender
- In a bowl, add eggs and 1 cup of heavy cream; whisk together
- Place ham, onions, broccoli, and cheese in a greased 9" pie plate or quiche pan
- Pour egg mixture over the meat and veggies
- Place in oven and bake for 35-40 mins
- Remove and let cool for about 5 mins before cutting and serving

Optional fillings include mushrooms, green or red peppers and jalapenos

Nutritional Information per serving
319 calories
26 g fat
5 g carbohydrates
1 g fiber
17 g protein

Deconstructed Eggrolls

6 servings

Prep time: 5 mins
Total time: 10 mins

Ingredients
1 lb ground pork
1 head cabbage, thinly sliced
1/2 medium onion, thinly sliced
1 tbsp sesame oil
1/4 cup soy sauce or liquid aminos
1 clove garlic, minced
1 tsp ground ginger
2 tbsp chicken broth
salt and pepper to taste
2 stalks green onion, for garnish

Directions
- Brown ground pork in a large pan or wok over medium heat
- Add sesame oil and onion to pan with browned ground pork; mix together and continue cooking over medium heat
- Add soy sauce, garlic, and ground ginger together in a small bowl and mix
- Once onions have browned, add sauce mixture to the pan
- Add cabbage mixture to the pan and toss to coat the vegetables; evenly distribute ingredients
- Add chicken broth to the pan and mix
- Continue cooking over medium heat for three mins, stirring frequently
- Garnish with salt, pepper, and green onion

Nutritional Information per serving
268 calories
18 g fat
10 g carbohydrates
4 g fiber
15 g protein

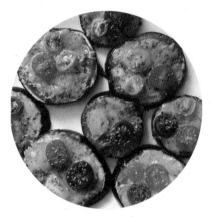

Eggplant Pizzas

2 servings (5 pieces per serving)

Prep time: 10 mins
Total time: 25 mins

Ingredients
1 eggplant, trimmed, cut in thick slices, skin on
1/2 tsp sea salt
3/4 cup low-sugar pizza sauce or marinara sauce
1/2 cup grated mozzarella cheese
1/3 cup baby spinach leaves
10 cherry tomatoes
1 tsp garlic olive oil (optional)
1 tsp dried oregano

Directions
- Preheat oven to 425° F
- Line baking sheet with parchment

paper and arrange eggplant slices on the sheet, making sure they don't overlap
- Sprinkle the sea salt on top; set aside for 10 mins
- Bake for 15 mins
- Remove baked eggplant slices from the oven, flip them over and switch the oven to broil mode
- For extra flavour and moisture, brush garlic olive oil on top of each eggplant slice
- Spread about 1 tbsp of pizza/marinara sauce over each eggplant slice
- Add baby spinach leaves, grated mozzarella cheese, and half cherry tomatoes (or toppings of your choice)
- Add sprinkle of dried oregano and return to oven, on broil, for 3-5 mins, or until the cheese is grilled and melted

Nutritional Information per slice
24 calories
0.6 g fat
2.6 g carbohydrates
1.2 g fiber
2.7 g protein

Fat Head Pizza Dough

1 Pizza Crust (8 slices)

Prep time: 5 mins
Total time: 20 mins

Ingredients
3/4 cup almond flour OR 1/2 cup coconut flour
1 1/2 cups shredded cheese
2 tbsp cream cheese
1 tbsp baking powder
1 egg

Directions
- Mix flour and baking powder together in a bowl; set aside
- In a separate bowl melt shredded cheese and cream cheese together in the microwave for 2 mins, stirring halfway through
- Add melted cheeses and egg to the flour mixture; combine well
- Place dough between two sheets of parchment paper and roll out with rolling pin
- Remove top sheet, pierce with a fork
- Bake for 12-15 mins at 425° F
- Remove from oven; add sauce, toppings, and additional cheese and bake another 5-10 mins

NOTE: You can also add spices of choice to flour mixture, if desired, e.g., 1/4 tsp garlic, onion powder, chili powder, pizza spice, and/or oregano. This dough is also great for pizza crust, pizza pockets, and calzones. If chilled after mixing, it's quite easy to work with.

Nutritional Information per full crust
200 calories
15 g fat
4.5 g carbohydrates
1.5 g fiber
11 g protein

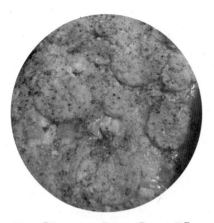

Daikon Au Gratin (Faux Scalloped Potatoes)

8 servings

Prep time:10 mins
Total time: 1 hr 15 mins

Ingredients
1/2 large daikon radish, thinly sliced, about 4 C
1 cup onions, thinly sliced
4 tbsp butter
1 cup heavy cream
2 cups shredded cheese
2 tbsp dried parsley
2 tbsp dried chives
1/2 tsp onion powder
1/2 tsp garlic powder
2 tsp pepper
1/4 cup Parmesan cheese

Directions
- Soak sliced daikon radish in cold, salted water for 20 mins; pat dry with paper towels
- Preheat oven to 325° F
- Arrange all sliced daikon in an ungreased 9x12" casserole dish
- Over medium heat, cook onion in butter until transparent, stirring occasionally (just a few mins)
- Add parsley, chives, garlic and onion powder and pepper; stir, just until bubbling; add cream and stir occasionally until heated through (about 5 mins)
- Remove from heat and add cheese; stir until cheese is melted and worked into the sauce
- Pour thickened liquid over the radishes
- Bake, covered, for 45 mins, or until cheese is golden and bubbly; sprinkle with 1/4 cup Parmesan cheese
- Bake for 10-20 mins uncovered to crust up the cheese slightly

Nutritional Information per serving
250 calories
22 g fat
4.6 g carbohydrates
0.3 g fiber
5.5 g protein

Faux-tato Salad
6 servings

Prep time: 20 mins
Total time: 2 hrs

1 head cauliflower, cut in pieces, and steamed
4 hard-boiled eggs
3/4 cup mayonnaise
1 small onion, chopped
salt and pepper to taste

- Chop steamed cauliflower and egg into small pieces
- Mix in remaining ingredients and chill before serving

Nutritional Information per serving
260 calories
23 g fat
7 g carbohydrates
2 g fiber
5.5 g protein

Fettuccini Alfredo Noodle and Sauce
1 serving

Prep time: 10 mins
Total time: 20 mins

Ingredients
For the noodles
2 eggs
1 oz cream cheese
pinch of salt
pinch of garlic powder
1/2 tsp pepper

For the sauce
1 oz mascarpone cheese
1 tbsp grated Parmesan cheese
1 tbsp butter OR 1 tbsp grated Parmesan cheese
2 oz cream cheese
2 tbsp heavy cream
1 tbsp butter

Directions
- Blend noodle ingredients in blender until smooth
- Pour into a greased 8x8" pan
- Bake at 325° F for 8 mins or until set (firm to touch)
- Remove and let cool for 5 mins
- Cut into 1/8 inch noodle strips
- To make the sauce add ingredients of your choice to a microwave-safe bowl and heat 30 secs; remove and whisk until smooth
- Coat pasta with the sauce; garnish with fresh parsley or basil

Nutritional Information per serving
486 calories
46 g fat
2.4 g carbohydrates
0.1 g fiber
18 g protein

Flax Crackers

1 serving

Prep time: 5 mins
Total time: 15 mins

Ingredients
1/2 cup ground flax seed
1/2 cup hot water
spices of choice, such as cocoa powder, cinnamon, cumin, garlic or onion powder, or Italian seasoning

Directions
- In a bowl mix flax seed, water, and seasoning of choice
- Spread out on a round pizza-like shape on microwavable plate lined with parchment paper
- Microwave in 2-3-min increments until crispy, roughly 6-8 mins depending on microwave

Nutritional Information per serving
420 calories
34 g fat
24 g carbohydrates
22 g fiber
14 g protein

Jalapeno Crisps

8 servings

Prep time: 15 mins
Total time: 25 mins

Ingredients
4 slices bacon
1 cup Parmesan cheese, finely shredded
1/2 cup shredded cheddar
1 jalapeno, thinly sliced
ground pepper

Directions
- Preheat oven to 375° F
- In a pan, over medium heat, cook bacon until crispy, about 8 mins; drain on a paper-towel lined plate, then chop
- Spoon about 1 tbsp Parmesan into a small mound on a large baking sheet and top with about 1 tbsp of cheddar cheese
- Carefully pat down cheeses and top with a jalapeno slice
- Top with bacon and season with pepper
- Repeat with remaining ingredients
- Bake until crispy and golden, about 12 mins
- Let cool slightly on pan before serving

Nutritional Information per serving
90 calories
7 g fat
0.4 g carbohydrates
0 g fiber
7 g protein

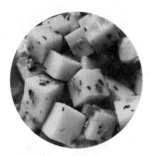

Jalapeno-marinated Mozzarella Cubes

6 servings

Prep time: 10 mins
Total time: 12 hrs & 10 mins

Ingredients
1 lb fresh mozzarella, cubed
1/2 cup olive oil
2 jalapenos, seeded and minced
1 tsp dried basil
1 tsp crushed red pepper
1 tsp garlic, minced
1 tsp Himalayan salt
1 tsp fresh ground pepper

Directions
- Place cubed cheese in a storage bowl
- Mix all remaining ingredients together in a separate bowl
- Pour mixture over cheese and mix to coat
- Cover and refrigerate for at least 12 hrs

Nutritional Information per serving
200 calories
15 g fat
3 g carbohydrates
0.1 g fiber
14 g protein

Jamaican Jerk Chicken

4 servings

Prep time: 1 hr
Total time: 1.5 hrs

1 lb chicken thighs
1 cup cauliflower
1 cup broccoli
1 cup green pepper
1 cup 35% cream

Marinade
1 tsp garlic powder
1 tsp onion powder
1 tsp ginger
1/2 tsp thyme
1/2 tsp cinnamon
1/2 tsp chili powder
1/2 tsp salt
1/2 tsp pepper
2 tbsp soy sauce
2 tbsp lime juice
1 tbsp rice vinegar

Directions
- Marinate chicken thighs minimum 1 hr
- Cook chicken thighs in butter or fat
- Add veggies
- Mix well and simmer 5 min
- Add milk/cream
- Mix well and simmer 10 mins

Nutritional Information per serving
460 calories
40 g fat
12 g carbohydrates
2 g fiber
30 g protein

Meatloaf
8 servings

Prep time: 5 mins
Total time: 1 hr

Ingredients
2 lb ground beef
1/2 cup ground flax seed
1/4 cup onion, diced
6 cloves garlic, minced
3 oz tomato paste
2 tbsp Worcestershire sauce
2 eggs
1 tbsp Italian seasoning
2 tsp sea salt
1 tsp pepper
1/3 cup low-sugar/sugar-free ketchup (optional)

Directions
- Preheat oven to 350° F
- Grease a 9x5" pan
- In a large bowl combine all ingredients, except the ketchup, together. Mix until well incorporated but do not overmix
- Transfer to the 9x5" pan
- Bake 30 mins
- If using spread ketchup on top of meatloaf and bake additional 35-45 mins, until cooked through
- Rest 10 mins before slicing

Nutritional Information per serving
375 calories
27 g fat
4.4 g carbohydrates
2.2 g fiber
27 g protein

Mock Sweet Potato Casserole with Pecan Topping
10 servings

Prep time: 5 mins
Total time: 35 mins

Ingredients
1 head cauliflower
1 cup mashed pumpkin
1/3 cup Sukrin Gold sweetener
3 eggs
1/2 tsp salt
4 tbsp butter
1 tsp cinnamon
1 tsp nutmeg
1/2 tsp ginger
1/4 tsp cloves

For the pecan topping
3 tbsp Sukrin Gold sweetener
2 tbsp coconut flour
3 tbsp almond flour
4 tbsp butter
3/4 cup chopped pecans

Directions
- Cut cauliflower into florets and steam until soft
- Combine steamed cauliflower, pumpkin, sweetener, eggs, salt, butter, cinnamon, nutmeg, ginger, and cloves in food processor or blender
- Purée until smooth
- Spread mashed cauliflower mixture into 2-quart or 11x17" casserole dish

Topping
- In medium bowl, mix together Sukrin Gold, coconut flour, and almond flour
- Cut in butter; stir in pecans
- Sprinkle pecan mixture over cauliflower mixture
- Bake at 325° F for 30 mins or until topping has browned

Nutritional Information per serving
200 calories
18 g fat
7G carbohydrates
3 g fiber
5 g protein

No-chop Chili
4 servings

Prep time: 5 mins
Total time: 15 mins

Ingredients
1 LB ground beef
1/2 cup salsa (low-sugar)
spices of choice
garlic powder, chili powder, cumin, onion powder

Directions
- Brown ground beef, add spices and salsa; cook through
- Serve with 2 tbsp full-fat sour cream and top with green onions and shredded cheese

Nutritional Information per serving
400 calories
29 g fat
8.5G carbohydrates
0.3 g fiber
30 g protein

Parmesan/Dill Cheese Chips
1 serving (15 chips)

Prep time: 5 mins
Total time: 10 mins

Ingredients
1/2 cup shredded mozzarella cheese
1 tbsp shredded Parmesan cheese
1 tbsp dill seed
sea salt for topping

Directions
- Preheat oven to 350° F
- Line baking sheet with parchment paper or silicone mat
- Place shredded mozzarella in mounds on paper
- Add Parmesan, dill, and sea salt to each mound
- Bake until desired crispiness

Nutritional Information per 15 chips
200 calories
14 g fat
6 g carbohydrates
0 g fiber
17 g protein

Loaded "Potato" Skins

3 servings (4 skins per serving)

Prep time: 25 mins
Total time: 1 hr

Ingredients
16 oz cauliflower (fresh or frozen)
1 cup shredded cheddar cheese, divided
2 tbsp heavy cream
1 egg
1 tbsp butter
3 slices bacon
8 tbsp sour cream
1/4 cup green onions
salt and pepper to taste

Directions
- Preheat oven to 375° F
- Steam cauliflower for 10 mins in microwave until tender; drain excess liquid
- Add cauliflower, 1/2 cup shredded cheese, heavy cream, butter, egg, salt and pepper to food processor and blend until smooth and creamy
- Using a silicone muffin tray OR a muffin tin sprayed with non-stick spray, spoon the cauliflower mixture into the bottom of each cup, pressing gently in the middle to form a well
- Bake for 35 mins until the "skins" are golden brown
- Cook bacon in the microwave until crispy; crumble
- Let skins cool for 10 mins before transferring to a lined baking sheet
- Sprinkle remaining shredded cheese evenly among the skins and top with crumbled bacon
- Return to oven for 5 mins until the cheese melts
- Top with sour cream and green onions

Nutritional Information per serving
324 calories
27 g fat
8 g carbohydrates
1 g fiber
15 g protein

Quesadillas

4 servings

Prep time: 10 mins
Total time: 30 mins

Ingredients
1 tbsp extra-virgin olive oil
1 bell pepper, sliced
1/2 yellow onion, sliced
1 tsp chili powder
salt and black pepper
3 cups shredded Monterey Jack
3 cups shredded cheddar
4 cups shredded chicken
1 avocado, thinly sliced
1 green onion, thinly sliced
Sour cream, for serving

Directions
- Preheat oven to 400° F and line two medium baking sheets with

parchment paper

- In a medium skillet over medium-high heat, heat oil; add bell pepper and onion; season with chili powder, salt, and pepper
- Cook until soft for 5 mins; transfer to a plate
- In a medium bowl, stir together cheeses
- Add 1 1/2 cups of cheese mixture into the centre of both prepared baking sheets
- Spread into an even layer and shape into a circle, the size of a flour tortilla
- Bake cheeses for 8-10 mins until melted and slightly golden around the edge
- Add onion-pepper mixture, shredded chicken, and avocado slices to one half of each
- Let cool slightly, then use the parchment paper and a small spatula to gently lift and fold one side of the cheese "tortilla" over the side with the fillings
- Return to oven to heat for 3-4 mins
- Repeat to make 2 more quesadillas
- Cut each quesadilla into quarters; garnish with green onion and sour cream before serving

Nutritional Information per serving
1000 calories
75 g fat
14 g carbohydrates
3.5 g fiber
74 g protein

Cauliflower Risotto
4 servings

Prep time: 5 mins
Total time: 25 mins

Ingredients
1/4 cup butter
8 oz mushrooms, chopped
2 cloves garlic, minced
Salt and pepper to taste
12 oz riced cauliflower
1/4 cup dry white wine
1/4-1/2 cup chicken broth
2-4 tbsp heavy cream
1/2 cup grated Parmesan cheese

Directions
- In a large sauté pan, heat butter over medium heat until melted and hot
- Add chopped mushrooms and garlic and sauté until mushrooms are tender and just turning golden brown; season with salt and pepper
- Reduce heat to medium low, add cauliflower, and toss to coat in the butter
- Add white wine and cook until the liquid has bubbled away
- Add broth a few tbsp at a time, stirring frequently and letting it evaporate each time
- When cauliflower is becoming tender, add a little more broth and a few tbsp cream
- Cover with lid and continue to cook, allowing the cauliflower to steam

...more

continued...

until tender; add a bit more broth and/or cream if needed
- Stir in the Parmesan and add salt and pepper to taste
- Serve with additional grated Parmesan as desired

Nutritional Information per serving
245 calories
19.7 g fat
5 g carbohydrates
2.3 g fiber
9.2 g protein

Simple Egg Salad
3 servings (1/2 cup each)

Prep time: 5 mins
Total time: 15 mins

Ingredients
6 eggs
2 tbsp mayo
1 tsp lemon juice
1/2 tsp salt
Add-ins: diced pickles, chili powder, or a small amount of finely diced red onion

Directions
- Place eggs in a pot and cover with water; bring to a boil and cook eggs 6-7 mins; let cool
- Peel and dice eggs
- Add all remaining ingredients and mix

- Serve on cloud bread, keto rolls, or lettuce leaves

Nutritional Information per serving
150 calories
12 g fat
1 g carbohydrates
0 g fiber
8 g protein

Simple Keto Crackers
4 servings

Prep time: 5 mins
Total time: 20 mins

Ingredients
2 cups almond flour
1/2 tsp salt
1 egg, beaten

Directions
- Preheat oven to 350° F
- Mix all ingredients
- Knead into dough; roll out and cut into crackers
- Prick centres with a fork
- Bake 15 mins

Nutritional Information per serving
98 calories
8.2 g fat
3.1 g carbohydrates
1.5 g fiber
4.6 g protein

Sloppy Joe Meat

6 servings (1/2 cup each)

Prep time: 5 mins
Total time: 30 mins

Ingredients
1 LB lean ground beef
1/2 cup diced green pepper
1/4 cup diced onion
1 clove garlic, minced
1/4 cup tomato paste
2 tbsp Sukrin Gold sweetener
1 tbsp yellow mustard
1 tsp red wine vinegar
2 tsp Worcestershire sauce
1 cup beef broth
1/2 tsp each of salt and pepper

Directions
- Chop green pepper and onion; mince garlic
- Place the ground beef in a frying pan and sauté
- When the meat is almost cooked through, stir in all the other ingredients, finishing with the broth
- Bring to a simmer; turn down to medium low and simmer uncovered for about 15 mins
- Serve on a Keto-friendly bun, over konjac rice, or in lettuce wraps

Nutritional Information per serving
233 calories
17 g fat
4 g carbohydrates
1 g fiber
15G protein

Keto Sour Cream and Chive Crackers

15 servings (1 serving = 4 crackers)

Prep time: 10 mins
Total time: 50 mins

Ingredients
1 3/4 cups mozzarella cheese, shredded
2 tbsp sour cream
1 egg
1/4 cup almond flour
1/4 cup coconut flour
2 tbsp chives
2 tbsp butter
1/8 tsp salt

Directions
- Preheat oven to 400° F
- Melt shredded mozzarella in a frying pan over medium heat (an also be done in a microwave)
- Remove from heat; add sour cream; stir until well combined
- In a mixing bowl add almond flour, coconut flour, egg, and chives to the cheese mixture; mix until well combined
- Wrap the dough in plastic wrap, then place in the fridge for 10- 15 mins
- Between 2 pieces of parchment paper, with a rolling pin roll the dough very thinly; remove the top piece of parchment paper
- Use a cookie cutter or a knife to cut out shapes

...more

continued...

- Place the shapes onto a baking sheet lined with parchment paper
- Brush the tops with the melted butter; sprinkle with salt
- Bake for 8-10 mins, watching them closely
- Place any dough scraps back in the fridge for another 10-15 mins before rolling out again

Nutritional Information per serving
85 calories
6.6 g fat
1.9 g carbohydrates
0.9 g fiber
4.1 g protein

Steak Bites

4 servings

Prep time: 10 mins
Total time: 3 hrs

Ingredients
1/2 cup soy sauce
1/3 cup olive oil
1/4 cup Worcestershire sauce
1 tsp minced garlic
2 tbsp dried basil
1 tbsp dried parsley
1 tsp black pepper
1-1/2 LB flat iron or top sirloin steak, cut in 1-inch pieces

Instructions
- Place all ingredients, except steak, in a large Ziploc bag; stir with a spoon to combine
- Drop steak pieces in and seal shut; shake gently to coat steak entirely in marinade
- Place bag in refrigerator to marinate for 3-24 hrs
- Heat large skillet over medium-high heat; heat skillet until it's very hot
- Remove steak pieces from marinade using a slotted spoon and place in hot skillet; discard marinade
- Cook steak according to your desired temperature; medium-well is about 3 mins
- Serve warm

Nutritional Information per serving
404 calories
30 g fat
6.7 g carbohydrates
0.8 g fiber
23.5 g protein

Stuffed Meatballs

16 meatballs (8 servings of 2 balls each)

Prep time: 10 mins
Total time: 30 mins

Ingredients
1 LB fresh hot Italian sausage
1 LB ground beef
2-3 mozzarella cheese sticks

1/2 cup Parmesan Cheese Whisps (crushed)
1 jar low sugar marinara sauce
8 oz mozzarella cheese
2 tbsp olive oil
1 tsp pink Himalayan salt
1 tsp black pepper
1 tsp dried oregano
1 tsp granulated garlic
1 tsp dried parsley
1 tsp crushed red pepper flakes (optional)

Directions
- Preheat the oven to broil (usually about 500° F)
- In a large mixing bowl combine beef with hot Italian sausage
- Add in the Crushed Parmesan Cheese Whisps, granulated garlic, salt, pepper, and oregano; combine well
- Slice the mozzarella cheese sticks into roughly ½-inch-long sections
- Oil an oven-safe pan with your choice of oil (avocado oil is usually preferred for high-heat applications like this as it has less of a tendency to smoke)
- Take a pinch of the meatball mixture and tuck one of the mozzarella cheese stick slices into the middle of it and roll into a ball
- Place meatballs in pan, and be sure to slide them back and forth a little bit when placing them in the pan to ensure that the bottom of the meatball is coated in oil to prevent them from sticking to the pan
- Place the pan of meatballs in the oven for 10-12 mins, or until the tops of the meatballs just begin to get a brown crisp on top
- Carefully remove the pan from the oven, and top the meatballs with the jar of marinara sauce, and 8 oz of shredded mozzarella cheese
- Place the pan back in the oven for about 5-7 mins, or until the mozzarella cheese on top is browned or bubbling to your liking
- Remove from the oven
- top with sprinkle of parsley and crushed red pepper flakes, if desired
- Serve alone or with zucchini noodles

Nutritional Information per serving
530 calories
39 g fat
6 g carbohydrates
0 g fiber
37 g protein

Philly Cheesesteak Filled Portobello Mushroom Caps

4 servings

Prep time: 10 mins
Total time: 30 mins

Ingredients
6 oz thinly sliced sirloin steak
1/8 tsp salt
pepper to taste
cooking spray
3/4 cup diced onion
3/4 cup diced green pepper
1/4 cup sour cream
2 tbsp mayonnaise
2 oz cream cheese, softened
3 oz shredded mild provolone cheese
(or cheese of your choice)
4 medium Portobello mushrooms,
with no cracks

Directions
- Preheat oven to 400° F
- Spray baking sheet with oil
- Gently remove the stems, scoop
  out the gills, and spray the tops of
  the mushrooms with oil; season
  with salt and fresh pepper
- Season steak with salt and pepper
  on both sides
- Spray large skillet with cooking
  spray and heat on high; let the pan
  get very hot then add the steak and
  cook on high heat about 1-1 1/2
  mins on each side, until cooked
  through
- Transfer to a cutting board and
  slice thinly; set aside
- Reduce heat to medium-low; spray
  with more oil and sauté onions and
  peppers 5-6 mins, until soft
- Combine all ingredients in a
  medium bowl
- Transfer to the mushroom caps,
  about 1/2 cup each
- Bake in the oven until the cheese
  is melted and the mushrooms are
  tender, about 20 mins

Nutritional Information (1 cap)
256 calories
16 g fat
10 g carbohydrates
4 g fiber
19 g protein

Stuffed Peppers

8 servings

Prep time: 5 mins
Total time: 1 hr

Ingredients
8 green peppers
1 LB ground beef
4 cups riced cauliflower
1 cup sliced mushrooms
2 cloves garlic, minced
1 cup low-sugar tomato sauce
1/2 tsp paprika
1/2 tsp rosemary
1/2 tsp oregano
1/2 tsp basil
1/2 tsp pepper

Directions
- Slice tops off green peppers and reserve; remove cores and seeds
- Steam peppers 7-8 mins; set aside
- In large bowl, combine riced cauliflower and herbs and mix well
- In large skillet, sauté onion, garlic, mushrooms, and ground beef over medium heat until fully cooked; stir into rice mixture
- Place green peppers in a baking dish
- Fill each pepper with rice/meat mixture and cover with reserved tops; additional mixture can be placed around the peppers
- Cover with foil and bake 1 hr at 350° F

Nutritional Information per serving
186 calories
6.8 g fat
18 g carbohydrates
4.8 g fiber
18 g protein

Bacon/Cream Cheese Stuffed Tenderloin

3 servings

Prep time: 20 mins
Total time: 50 mins

Ingredients
1- 1 1/2 LB pork tenderloin, silverskin removed

2 slices thick-cut bacon, diced
4 oz cream cheese, softened
3 oz manchego OR Parmesan cheese, grated
1/2 cup baby spinach leaves

Balsamic Caramelized Onions
1 large red onion, cut into rings
2 tbsp butter
2 tbsp balsamic vinegar
1-2 tbsp mesquite seasoning

Directions
- Preheat skillet over medium-high heat; add the bacon pieces and cook until the fat is rendered, and the bacon pieces are crisp
- Remove bacon pieces to a paper towel to drain and leave the bacon fat in the pan
- Add butter and sliced red onions; cook for about 20 mins over medium heat, stirring occasionally, until onions have darkened considerably in colour
- Reduce heat to low and stir in the balsamic vinegar
- Remove onions from the pan and set aside
- Place the pork tenderloin on a large cutting board; remove any excess fat or silverskin from the exterior of the tenderloin
- Butterfly the pork tenderloin by using long strokes of your knife along the side of the tenderloin about ½ inch above the cutting board; keep the slices parallel to the cutting board and roll open the

...more

continued...

tenderloin while slicing
- Spread the softened cream cheese on top of the butterflied tenderloin; sprinkle with the shredded manchego or Parmesan cheese, caramelized onions, baby spinach leaves, and bacon pieces
- Starting with the edge of the pork tenderloin that was the inside (before slicing open) begin tightly rolling the tenderloin back up
- Tie the roll together with butcher's twine every inch to inch and a half until the roll is nice and bound (NOTE: you can also use toothpicks to close up the meat if you do not have twine)
- Season the pork tenderloin liberally with mesquite seasoning
- Grill over indirect, medium-high heat (about 375° F) for approximately 20-25 mins or until the internal temperature of the tenderloin is 145° F in the thickest part of the meat; turn tenderloin every 5 mins while cooking
- Allow the tenderloin to rest at least 5 mins before removing the butcher's twine
- Slice the tenderloin into 1-inch-thick rounds

Nutritional Information per serving
200 calories
11 g fat
1 g carbohydrates
0.3 g fiber
20 g protein

Taco Bites
20 bites

Prep time: 10 mins
Total time: 30 mins

Ingredients
1 LB ground beef
3 tbsp homemade taco seasoning (see p. 116)
2 tbsp butter
6 eggs
4 oz shredded cheese, divided
1/2 cup salsa (low-sugar)

Directions
- Sauté ground beef until browned; add taco seasoning; cook completely and let cool
- Preheat oven to 350° F
- In a bowl whisk eggs; add cooked ground beef, salsa, and 2 oz shredded cheese
- Fill silicone muffin moulds about 3/4 full with mixture and top with remaining cheese
- Bake 15-20 mins
- Serve with salsa and full-fat sour cream

Nutritional Information per bite
86 calories
5.9 g fat
0.1 g carbohydrates
0 g fiber
7.9 g protein

Taco Casserole

6 servings

Prep time: 5 mins
Total time: 45 mins

Ingredients
1 LB ground beef
1/4 cup chopped onion
1 jalapeno, minced
2 tbsp homemade taco seasoning
(see p. 116)
1/4 cup water
2 oz cream cheese
1/4 cup salsa
4 eggs
1 tbsp hot sauce
1/4 cup heavy whipping cream
1/2 cup grated cheddar
1/2 cup grated pepperjack/habenero
cheese

Directions
- Preheat oven to 350° F
- Spray 8x8" baking dish with non-
  stick spray
- Brown ground beef in a large skillet
  over medium heat
- Add onion and jalapeno to the beef
  and cook until onion is translucent;
  drain grease
- Stir in taco seasoning and water
  and cook for 5 mins
- Add cream cheese and salsa and
  stir to combine
- Crack eggs in a medium mixing
  bowl and whisk together with hot
  sauce and heavy cream
- Pour meat mixture into the

prepared baking dish and top with
egg mixture
- Sprinkle with cheese and bake for
  30 mins or until eggs are set
- Cool 5 mins before cutting
  and serving

Nutritional Information per serving
406 calories
28 g fat
5 g carbohydrates
1 g fiber
30 g protein

Tomato Soup

4 servings

Prep time: 5 mins
Total time: 10 mins

Ingredients
1 can tomato paste
1 cup heavy whipping cream
3/4 cup shredded cheese
1/4-1/2 cup water (depending on
how thick you like it)
1 tsp oregano
1 tsp garlic, minced
salt and pepper to taste
green onion or parsley to garnish

Directions
- Place tomato paste, garlic, and
  oregano in a pot over medium heat
- Add heavy cream and bring to a
  boil while whisking
- Add cheese little by little until it

...more

continued...

starts to thicken; add water and cook additional 4-5 mins

Nutritional Information per serving
407 calories
33 g fat
8 g carbohydrates
2.6 g fiber
12.5 g protein

Tortilla Chips

8 servings

Prep time: 10 mins
Total time: 15 mins

Ingredients
2 cups shredded mozzarella
3/4 cup almond flour
2 tbsp psyllium husk powder
pinch salt
Optional: 1/4 tsp each garlic powder/onion powder/paprika

Directions
- Preheat oven to 350° F
- Melt mozzarella cheese in microwave, 90 sec-2 mins
- Add almond flour and psyllium husk, and salt and spices, if using
- Stir until combined, then knead until you have a smooth dough
- Separate the dough into 2 balls

and roll out between 2 sheets of baking/parchment paper
- Roll out as thinly as possible; the thinner they are, the crispier your tortilla chips will be
- Cut into triangles using a pizza cutter and spread out on a sheet of baking paper so the tortilla chips don't touch
- Bake 6-8 mins or until browned on the edges; baking time will depend on the thickness of the tortilla chips

Nutritional Information per serving
143 calories
9.2 g fat
4.8 g carbohydrates
2.9 g fiber
8.3 g protein

Zucchini Fries

2 servings

Prep time: 10 mins
Total time: 30 mins

Ingredients
2 medium zucchinis
1/4 cup grated Parmesan cheese
1 egg, whisked
1/2 tsp garlic powder
1/2 tsp pepper

Directions
- Preheat oven to 425° F
- Remove ends from zucchini and cut into strips resembling fries
- Prepare two bowls, 1 with whisked egg mixed with spices and 1 with

Parmesan cheese
- Dip your zucchini fries into egg then into cheese, coating well
- Place on baking sheet lined with parchment paper
- Bake 20 mins, flipping after 10 mins

Nutritional Information per serving
185 calories
11 g fat
6 g carbohydrates
2 g fiber
16 g protein

Zucchini Ravioli
9 servings

Prep time: 10 mins
Total time: 35 mins

Ingredients
1 tbsp olive oil
4 zucchinis
4 cups baby spinach
2 cloves garlic, minced
3/4-1 cup ricotta cheese
1/3 cup shredded Parmesan cheese
1 cup marinara sauce (low sugar)
3/4 cup sliced mozzarella cheese

Directions
- Preheat oven to 350° F
- Peel zucchini into strips with vegetable peeler or knife; make about 36-40 strips equaling 9-10 raviolis

- Sauté spinach in olive oil and garlic
- Add ricotta to spinach and mix until coated
- Layer zucchini strips, two across and two over top in the shape of a number symbol (#)
- Add spinach/ricotta mixture in centre (roughly 1 tbsp) and fold zucchini; repeat until all zucchini and mixture is used
- Place raviolis folded side down into a greased casserole dish; top with marinara sauce and mozzarella; sprinkle with Parmesan cheese and salt and pepper
- Bake 20-25 mins

Nutritional Information per ravioli
99 calories
7 g fat
3.2 g carbohydrates
0.6 g fiber
4.9 g protein

THE KETO SOLUTION

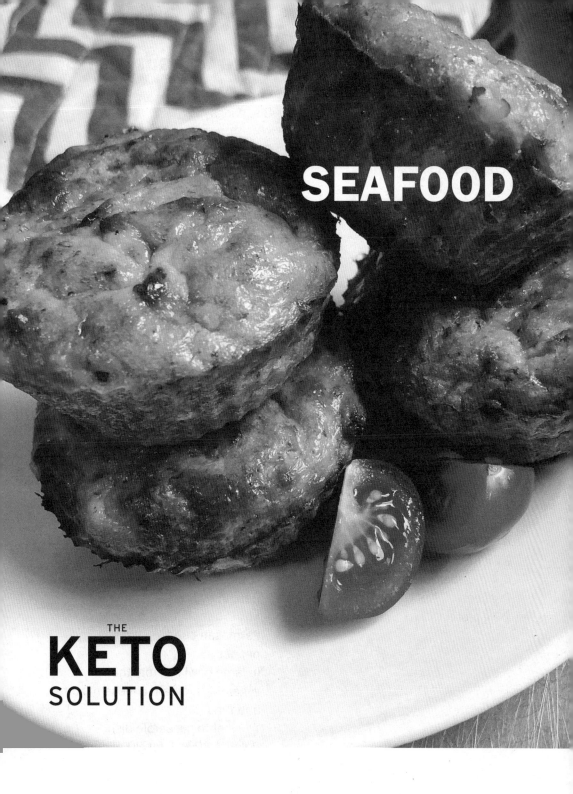

SEAFOOD

Fried Haddock with Garlic Aioli

2 servings

Prep time: 5 mins
Total time: 30 mins

Ingredients
8 oz fresh haddock
2 tbsp bacon fat

Aioli
1/2 cup mayonnaise
1 clove garlic, pressed
1 tbsp lemon juice
Salt and pepper to taste

Directions
- Mix aioli ingredients until well combined and refrigerate
- Pan-fry haddock in bacon fat until you can easily break it apart with a fork

Nutritional Information per serving
445 calories
37 g fat
4.4 g carbohydrates
0 g fiber
22 g protein

Keto Creamy Tuna Casserole

8 servings

Prep time: 5 mins
Total time: 50 mins

Ingredients
1/2 cup fresh grated Parmesan cheese
1 tbsp lemon juice
1-2 tbsp onion and chive dip spice
1/2 cup sour cream
1 pkg cream cheese
4 tbsp melted butter
1 medium red pepper, chopped
1 medium zucchini, chopped
1 small head cabbage, shredded
3 cans tuna, drained
salt and pepper to taste

Directions
- Fry cabbage in 2 tbsp butter until tender
- Fry red pepper and zucchini in 2 tbsp butter
- In glass bowl soften cream cheese in the microwave
- Beat in sour cream
- Mix in lemon juice, dip mix, Parmesan cheese, and salt and pepper
- In large bowl mix together vegetables, cream cheese mixture, and tuna
- Transfer to casserole dish
- Bake at 325° F for 30 mins

Nutritional Information per serving
297 calories
20 g fat
14 g carbohydrates
3 g fiber
18 g protein

Linda's Salmon Delight

2 servings

Prep time: 30 mins
Total time: 30 mins

Ingredients
1 can salmon, drained
1 cup diced fresh mushrooms
1 small onion, diced
1 cup finely chopped celery
1/2 cup whipping cream
3/4 cup fresh shredded Parmesan
1/2 cup grated mozzarella
3 tbsp butter
salt and pepper to taste
1 cup cooked cauliflower

Directions
- Sauté mushrooms, onions, and celery in butter
- Add salmon, cream, cheeses, and salt and pepper
- Heat until cheese is melted and serve over cooked cauliflower

Nutritional Information per serving
707 calories
56.5 g fat
9.5 g carbohydrates
3.5 g fiber
36 g protein

Salmon Cakes

14 servings

Prep time: 10 mins
Total Time: 40 mins

Ingredients
1 LB fresh salmon filet
3 tbsp olive oil
2 tbsp butter
1 tsp garlic salt (or to taste)
Black pepper, to taste
1 medium yellow onion, finely diced to make 1 C
1/2 red bell pepper, seeded and diced
1 cup finely crushed pork rinds
2 large eggs, lightly beaten
3 tbsp mayonnaise
1 tsp Worcestershire sauce
1/4 tsp black pepper
1/4 cup parsley, finely minced

Directions
- Preheat oven to 425° F
- Line rimmed baking sheet with parchment paper
- Place salmon in the centre, skin side down; drizzle with 1 tbsp olive oil and season with garlic salt and black pepper
- Bake uncovered for 10-15 min (depending on thickness), or just until cooked through
- Remove from oven, cover with foil, and rest 10 min
- Flake salmon with 2 forks, discarding skin and any bones,
...more

continued...

- then set aside and cool to room temp
- Heat a medium skillet over medium heat with 1 tbsp olive oil and 1 tbsp butter
- Add onion and bell pepper and sauté until golden and softened (7-9 mins); remove from heat
- In large mixing bowl combine flaked salmon, cooked pepper and onion, pork rinds, eggs, mayonnaise, Worcestershire sauce, garlic salt, black pepper, and chopped parsley; stir to combine
- Form into patties (about a heaping tbsp each) and mould with your hands into patties 2" wide by 1/3 to 1/2" thick
- In a clean non-stick pan, heat 1 tbsp oil and 1 tbsp butter until hot; add salmon patties in a single layer
- Sauté for 3-4 min per side or until golden brown and cooked through; if salmon patties brown too fast, reduce heat
- Remove finished patties to a plate lined with paper towel, and repeat with oil, butter, and salmon cakes

Nutritional Information per salmon cake
180 calories
14.5 g fat
1 g carbohydrates
0.3 g fiber
11.5 g protein

Simple Tuna Salad
2 servings (1/2 cup each)

Prep/total time: 5 mins

Ingredients
1 cup tuna (2 cans, drained)
3 tbsp mayo
1 tsp dried onion flakes
salt and pepper to taste
Optional add-ins: diced pickles, garlic powder, dill seed

Directions
-Mix all ingredients in a bowl
-Serve on cloud bread, Keto rolls or lettuce leaves

Nutritional Information per serving
208 calories
15.7 g fat
1.7 g carbohydrates
0.6 g fiber
15 g protein

Sushi Rolls

2 servings (1/2 roll)

Prep time: 10 mins
Total time: 10 mins

Ingredients
4 oz smoked salmon, sugar-free
3 tbsp cream cheese
1 oz avocado
1 oz English cucumber
1 sheet seaweed
1/2 tsp sesame seeds
1/2 chopped green onion
1 tbsp coconut aminos
1 tsp chili mayo (optional)
1 tsp wasabi (optional)

Directions
- Slice English cucumber on the diagonal, and then thinly slice each section into approximately 1/8-inch-thick strips
- Cut the avocado into slices that are approximately 1/8 inch thick
- Cut about a ½-inch strip of cream cheese off the block lengthwise; cut that in half lengthwise
- Place sheet of seaweed on parchment paper
- Take thin slices of the smoked salmon and place it evenly across the seaweed
- Put the cream cheese, cucumber, and avocado near the bottom edge of the sushi, about 1/2 to 1 inch from the edge
- Use the parchment paper to help you roll the sushi; once you get it started you should be able to finish rolling by hand
- Use a very SHARP knife to cut the sushi; the seaweed can be difficult to cut otherwise
- Cut into 8 to 10 pieces and serve with a small amount of coconut aminos (a soy sauce alternative) and optionally some chili mayo and/or wasabi if you like it spicy
- Top with sesame seeds and green onion for a finishing flavour

Nutritional Information per serving
190 calories
14 g fat
4 g carbohydrates
1 g fiber
15 g protein

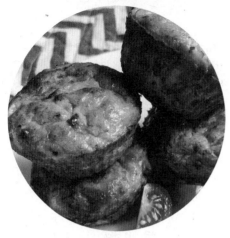

Tuna Muffins

6 servings

Ingredients
1 can of tuna, drained
1/2 cup mayo
2 eggs
2 baby dill pickles, chopped
1 tbsp no-sugar-added ketchup
2 cups grated cheddar cheese
salt and pepper to taste

Directions
- Preheat oven to 350° F
- Mix all ingredients together in a bowl
- Place in silicone muffin moulds
- Bake 20 mins

Nutritional Information per muffin
230 calories
11.3 g fat
2.2 g carbohydrates
0 g fiber
7.7 g protein

Tuna Melts

6 servings

Prep time: 5 mins
Total time: 25 mins

Ingredients
1 can tuna, drained
1/2 cup shredded cheese
1/4 cup mayo
4 tbsp sour cream
2 eggs
salt and pepper to taste

Directions
- Preheat oven to 350° F
- Mix all ingredients together in a bowl
- Place in silicone muffin moulds
- Bake 20 mins

Nutritional Information per serving
173 calories
14 g fat
0.8 g carbohydrates
0 g fiber
10.9 g protein

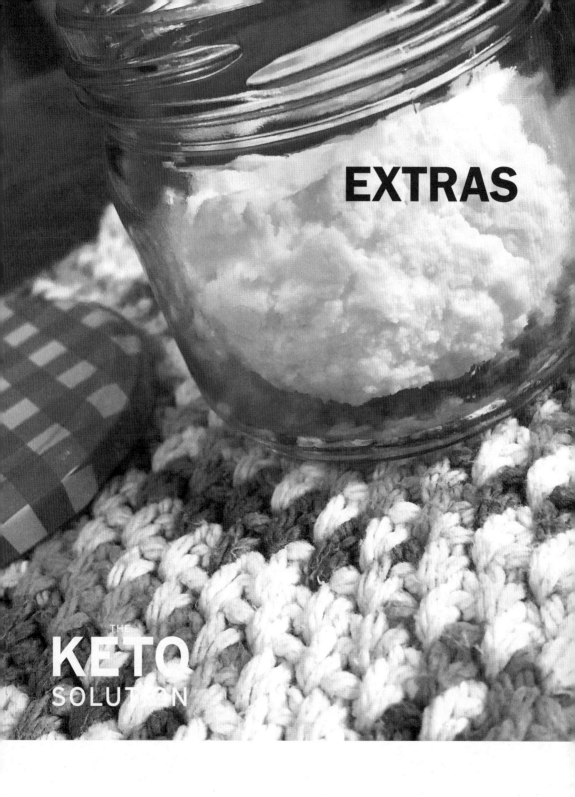

EXTRAS

KETO
SOLUTION

Creamy Alfredo Sauce

6 servings

Prep time: 5 mins
Total time: 10 mins

Ingredients
8 oz cream cheese, softened
3/4 cup heavy cream
2 oz freshly grated Parmesan cheese
1/4 tsp pepper
1/2 tsp garlic powder
salt, to taste
pinch of fresh parsley, minced (optional)

Directions
- In a medium saucepan, heat cream cheese on medium-low heat, stirring until melted and smooth
- Gradually blend in cream until smooth
- Stir in Parmesan and seasonings; cook and stir over low heat until smooth and creamy, thinning with water until thick but pourable
- Serve over chicken, vegetables, or other dishes
- Do not freeze

Nutritional Information
258 calories
24.9 g fat
1.8 g carbohydrates
0 g fiber
4.8 g protein

Avocado Dressing

6 servings

2 avocados, cubed
juice from 2 limes
1/4 cup olive oil (amount depends on desired consistency)
1 clove garlic, pressed
10 drops Stevia
salt and pepper
sprinkle of homemade taco seasoning (see p. 116)
1 cup chopped cilantro (or to taste)

Directions
- Combine all ingredients except olive oil. Whisk in olive oil until dressing has the right consistency

Nutritional Information per serving
165 calories
16.5 g fat
5.8 g carbohydrates
3.8 g fiber
1.2 g protein

Baked Broccoli Balls with Lemon Garlic Yogurt Sauce

3 servings

Prep time: 10 mins
Total time: 40 mins

Ingredients
Broccoli balls
2 cups (packed) roughly chopped soft cooked broccoli (well-drained)
1/4 cup crushed pork rinds
1/4 cup grated Parmesan cheese
2 eggs
3/4 cup shredded cheese of choice
2 shallots, finely sliced
2 cloves garlic, minced
1/4 tsp salt
Black pepper
Olive oil spray

Lemon garlic yogurt sauce
2/3 cup plain full-fat yogurt
Zest of 1/2 lemon
1 tbsp lemon juice
1/2 garlic clove, minced
1 tsp extra virgin olive oil
Salt and pepper, to taste

Directions
Broccoli balls
- Preheat oven to 350° F
- Line tray with parchment paper
- Place all ingredients (except oil spray) in a bowl; mix well to combine, mashing up the broccoli as you go
- Scoop up a heaped tbsp; press in firmly; form into a ball; place on tray
- Repeat with remaining mixture; should make 15-18 balls
- Spray with oil then bake for 25 mins, or until surface is slightly crisp and golden
- Serve with lemon yogurt sauce, or sugar-free/no-sugar-added ketchup

Lemon garlic yogurt sauce
- Mix ingredients together; set aside for at least 20 mins

Nutritional Information per serving
374 calories
15 g fat
9 g carbohydrates
6 g fiber
19.5 g protein

BBQ Sauce

6 servings

Prep time: 5 mins
Total time: 15 mins

Ingredients
1 cup apple cider vinegar
1/4 cup low/sugar-free ketchup
1/2 tsp garlic powder
1/2 tsp onion powder
1 tsp paprika
1/2 tsp ground cumin
1/2 tsp sea salt
2-3 drops liquid Stevia

Directions
- In a saucepan mix all ingredients together and heat until warm and fully mixed

Nutritional Information per serving
16 calories
0 g fat
0 g carbohydrates
0.2 g fiber
0 g protein

Dill Dip

Makes 2 C

Prep time: 10 mins
Total time: 1 hr (chill time)

Ingredients
8 oz cream cheese
8 oz full-fat sour cream
2 tbsp finely chopped green onion
2 tbsp chopped fresh dill OR 2 tsp dried dill
1/4 tsp salt

Directions
- In a medium bowl mix all ingredients with electric mixer until fluffy
- Cover and chill for 1 hr
- Serve with chicken wings or veggies

Option: You can also change this recipe to creamy blue cheese by preparing as above but omitting the dill and salt and adding 2 oz of crumbled blue cheese and 1/3 cup of finely chopped walnuts (this will change nutritional values)

Nutritional Information (per 1 tbsp)
55 calories
5 g fat
1 g carbohydrates
0 g fiber
1 g protein

Jill's Donair Sauce

6 servings

Prep time: 5 mins
Total time: 10 mins

1 cup 35% whipping cream
3 tsp garlic powder
3 tbsp vinegar
3 tbsp granular sweetener
4 drops liquid Stevia

Directions
- Place all ingredients in a mixer and mix on low for 5 mins to dissolve before turning it up to high to whip until thick
- Play with garlic and sweetener to your taste

Note: Make sure you buy gluten-free donair meat!

Nutritional Information per serving
125 calories
13 g fat
14.5 g carbohydrates
0 g fiber
1 g protein

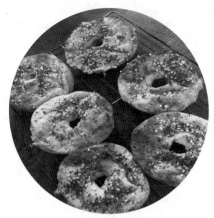

Everything Bagel Seasoning

5 servings

Prep/total time: 5 mins

Ingredients
2 tbsp poppy seeds
2 tbsp white sesame seeds
1 1/2 tbsp minced, dried onion
1 tbsp minced, dried garlic
1/2 tbsp sea salt

Directions
- Add all ingredients together in a jar; shake to combine

NOTE: This seasoning can be used as bagel seasoning or to top scrambled eggs, avocado, or salads

Nutritional Information per serving
48 calories
3 g fat
3.9 g carbohydrates
1.5 g fiber
1.5 g protein

Greek Salad Dressing

Makes 350 mL

Prep/total time: 5 mins

3/4 cup olive oil
1/2 cup apple cider vinegar
1 tbsp sugar-free pancake syrup
1 tsp prepared mustard
1 tbsp Greek spice mix

Directions
- Mix ingredients together in a jar and shake well

Nutritional Information per 2 tbsp
120 calories
13.5 g fat
0.3 g carbohydrates
0.3 g fiber
0 g protein

Guacamole

4 servings

Prep time: 5 mins
Total time: 10 mins

Ingredients
2-3 ripe avocados
1-2 garlic cloves
1 lime, juiced
2 tbsp olive oil
1/2 white onion
1/2 cup fresh cilantro
1 tomato, diced
salt and pepper

Directions
- Peel avocados and mash with a fork; grate or chop the onion finely; squeeze the lime and pour in the juice
- Add tomato, olive oil, and finely chopped cilantro; add salt and pepper and blend well

Tip: For even faster guacamole, crush 2-3 avocados with a fork, add 2 tbsp sour cream, lime juice, and salt and pepper

Nutritional Information per serving
262 calories
13.6 g fat
30 g carbohydrates
9 g fiber
6 g protein

Honey Mustard Dressing

Makes 280 mL

Prep time/total time: 5 mins

Ingredients
1/2 cup full-fat sour cream
1/4 cup water
1/4 cup Dijon mustard
1 tbsp apple cider vinegar
1 tbsp sweetener

Directions
- Combine all ingredients in a bowl, whisking together
- Store in refrigerator for up to two weeks in a mason jar or airtight container

Nutritional Information per 2 tbsp
33 calories
2.5 g fat
0.5 g carbohydrates
0 g fiber
0.4 g protein

Italian Dressing

Makes 500 mL

Prep time/total time: 10 mins

Ingredients
1 cup light-tasting olive oil
3/4 cup red wine vinegar
1 clove garlic, minced
2 tbsp Dijon mustard
2 tbsp dried minced onion
1 1/2 tsp Italian seasoning
1 tsp crushed red pepper flakes
1 tsp sea salt, or to taste

Directions
- Combine all ingredients in a mason jar with lid; shake until well combined
- Chill

Nutritional Information per 2 tbsp
125 calories
13.5 g fat
0.4 g carbohydrates
0 g fiber
0 g protein

Homemade Taco Seasoning

Makes approximately 65 mL (13 tsp)

2 tbsp chili powder
1/2 tsp garlic powder
1/2 tsp onion powder
1/2 tsp chili flakes
1/2 tsp dried oregano
1/2 tsp paprika
1 tbsp cumin
2 tsp sea salt
2 tsp pepper

Directions
- Mix all ingredients and store in airtight container or mason jar

Nutritional Information per 1 tsp
8 calories
0.3 g fat
1.3 g carbohydrates
0 g fiber
0 g protein

Mason Jar Homemade Butter

1/2 cup serving

Prep/Total time: 12 mins

Ingredients
Mason jar (16 OZ)
1 cup heavy cream (38% MF)
cold water

Directions
- Pour heavy cream into the mason jar, filling it halfway; screw on the lid
- Shake mason jar for approximately 5-7 mins; after the first 2 mins you'll have whipped cream
- Keep shaking until you hear that a lump has formed inside, and shake an additional 30-60 secs after that
- Remove solids from the jar; remaining liquid is buttermilk to keep or discard
- Place solids into a small bowl
- Pour cold water over the butter and use your hands to squish it into a ball
- Discard water and repeat rinsing twice
- At this point you have butter; you can choose to add in seasonings such as salt, herbs, or garlic

Nutritional Information per serving
410 calories
44 g fat
3 g carbohydrates
0 g fiber
2 g protein

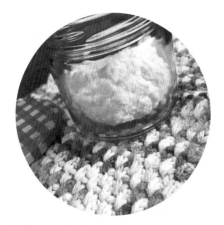

Keto Homemade Mayo

25 servings

Prep time/Total time: 10 mins

Ingredients
1 large egg
1 cup extra light-tasting olive oil
2-3 tsp lemon/lime juice OR apple cider vinegar
salt to taste

NOTE: You can also add alternative spices such as dill/garlic/chili powder to your liking

Directions
- Mix all ingredients together with immersion blender
- Store in mason jar in refrigerator for up to a month

Nutritional information (per 1 tbsp serving)
80 calories
9.2 g fat
0.1 g carbohydrates
0.3 g protein
0 g fiber

Parmesan Cream Cheese Dip

2 cups (12 servings)

Prep time: 10 mins
Total time: 2 hrs

Ingredients
8 oz cream cheese, softened
1 cup mayonnaise
1 tbsp lemon juice
2 tbsp onion/chive dip spice
1/4 tsp white pepper
sea salt to taste
1/2 cup shredded fresh Parmesan cheese

Directions
- Beat cream cheese and mayonnaise until smooth. Mix in remaining ingredients and chill for a few hrs.
- Serve warm or cold

Nutritional Information per serving (approximately 2.5 tbsp)
159 calories
15 g fat
2.3 g carbohydrates
2.4 g protein
0 g fiber

Protein Bounty Balls

25 balls

Prep time: 20 mins
Total time: 2.5 hrs

2 cups shredded coconut, unsweetened
1/2 cup vanilla protein powder, unsweetened
2 tbsp coconut flour
1/3 cup coconut oil, melted
1/3 cup full-fat coconut cream
2 tbsp Mrs. Butterworth's sugar-free maple syrup
3/4-1 cup Krisda sugar-free chocolate chips

Directions:
- Mix all ingredients, except the chocolate, together in a large bowl
- Roll into 25 balls
- Freeze to set, roughly 1-2 hrs
- Melt chocolate in microwave in 30-sec bursts and add 1 tbsp coconut oil
- Whisk until smooth
- Line a cookie sheet with parchment paper
- Dip balls into chocolate, place on sheet
  Freeze to set, about 10-15 mins
- Store in fridge or freezer

Nutritional Information per ball
86 calories
7.8 g fat
1.7 g carbohydrates
2 g fiber
2 g protein

Bacon/Jalapeno Snack Dip

1 serving

Prep time: 5 mins
Total time: 5 mins

Ingredients
2 oz cream cheese
2 tbsp shredded cheese of choice
1 tbsp jalapenos or pickles
1-2 strips bacon

Directions
- Cook 1-2 strips of bacon in microwave on high for 2-3 mins (depending on oven) or until desired crispiness; crumble
- Melt cheeses together in microwave
- Add remaining ingredients and mix

Nutritional Information (includes 2 strips of bacon)
442 calories
41 g fat
2.9 g carbohydrates
0.2 g fiber
14.6 g protein

Spinach Dip

4 servings

Prep time: 5 mins
Total time: 25 mins

Ingredients
5 oz cream cheese
4 cups baby spinach, finely chopped
1 tbsp butter
1/4 tsp garlic powder
1/4 tsp salt
1/4 tsp black pepper
1/3 cup heavy cream
1/8 tsp nutmeg (optional)
1/2 cup artichoke hearts, chopped
1 cup mozzarella cheese
1/4 cup Parmesan cheese, optional

Directions
- Melt butter in a saucepan
- Add chopped spinach; cook for 2 mins, until wilted
- Add salt, pepper, garlic, and nutmeg
- Add cream cheese; with the heat on low, incorporate cream cheese into the spinach
- Add cream and artichoke hearts
- Mix in half of the mozzarella cheese
- Transfer to a small oven-safe baking dish
- Top with remaining mozzarella and Parmesan cheese
- Bake for 20 mins, until the cheese is bubbly

Nutritional Information per serving
336 calories
29 g fat
6.2 g carbohydrates
1.2 g fiber
12 g protein

Coconut Butter

16 servings of 1 tbsp

Prep time: 10 mins
Total time: 10 mins

4 cups shredded unsweetened coconut
1 pinch sea salt
½ tsp vanilla
1 tsp erythritol/Stevia sweetener (optional)

Directions
- Place coconut in food processor and mix until "butter" forms (can take up to 10 mins)
- Mix in remaining ingredients
- Can be stored at room temperature for up to 2 weeks

Nutritional Information per serving
100 calories
10 g fat
4 g carbohydrates
2 g fiber
1 g protein

Trail Mix

16 servings

Prep time: 10 mins
Total time: 10 mins

1 cup roasted salted almonds
1 cup roasted salted pecans
1 cup macadamia nuts
1 cup peanuts
1 cup pistachios
1 cup keto/grain free granola
1 cup unsweetened coconut
1 cup sugar free chocolate chips
(Lily's or Krisda brand)

Directions
- Place coconut in food processor
  and mix until "butter" forms (can
  take up to 10 mins)
- Mix in remaining ingredients
- Can be stored at room temperature
  for up to 2 weeks

Nutritional Information per serving
(1/2 cup)
293 calories
27 g fat
17 g carbohydrates
2 g fiber
10 g protein

Cheesecake on-the-Go

5 servings of 2 tbsp

1 block cream cheese, softened
1/2 cup whipping cream
1/4 cup erythritol/Stevia sweetener
1 tsp vanilla

Directions
- Beat until well combined and store
  in refrigerator. May be used as a
  treat on its own, or can also be
  topped with berries, granola, etc.
  May also be used as a frosting.

Nutritional Information per serving
(2 tbsp)
200 calories
20 g fat
2.5 g carbohydrates
0 g fiber
3.5 g protein

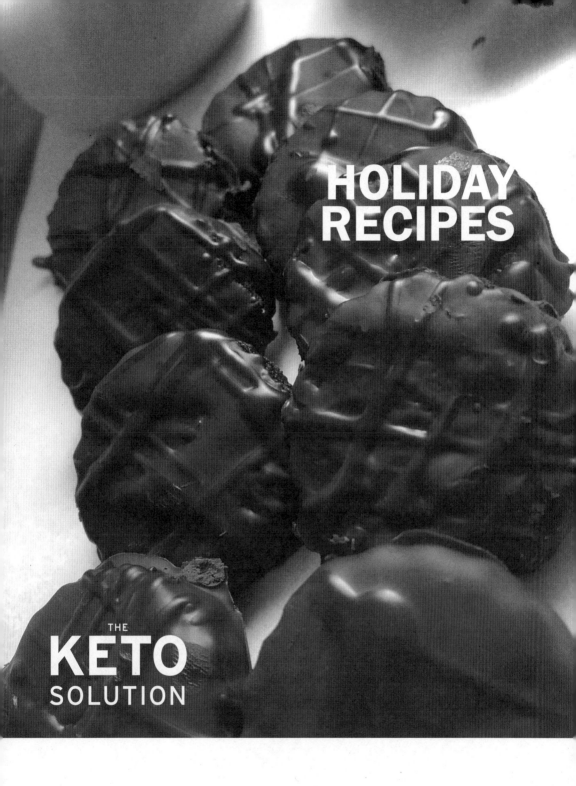

HOLIDAY
RECIPES

THE
KETO
SOLUTION

Cream Cheese Cookies

18 cookies

Prep time: 5 mins
Total time: 5 mins

1 block cream cheese, softened
1/2 cup butter, softened
1 tbsp vanilla
2 eggs
2 1/2 cups almond flour
1/2 cup no-calorie/no-carb sweetener

Directions
- Preheat oven to 350° F
- Blend cream cheese, butter, eggs, vanilla
- Add flour and sweetener; blend well
- Drop onto parchment-lined baking sheet
- Bake 15 mins

Nutritional Information per cookie
185 calories
18 g fat
4 g carbohydrates
1.7 g fiber
5 g protein

Almond Flour Butter Cookies

6 cookies

Prep time: 10 mins
Total time: 20 mins

1 cup of almond flour
1/4 cup erythritol sweetener
3 tbsp softened salted butter
1/2 tsp vanilla extract

Directions
- Preheat oven to 350° F
- Line a baking sheet with parchment paper
- Combine all ingredients in a mixing bowl and mix; it will look crumbly at first but will form a ball
- Form 1-inch balls (can use a small ice cream scoop)
- Flatten the balls with a folk in criss --cross pattern
- Bake at 350° F for 8-10 mins until golden brown at the edges
- Cookies will be very soft when they come out of the oven but will harden when cool to be just like shortbreads!

Nutritional Information per cookie
160 calories
15 g fat
4 g carbohydrates
1.7 g fiber
2 g protein

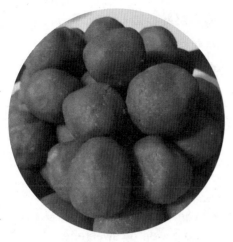

Nutritional Information per ball
115 calories
10.5 g fat
4 g carbohydrates
1 g fiber
2.5 g protein

Cherry Cheesecake Fat Bombs

12 fat bombs

Prep time: 20 mins
Total time: 2 hrs

1 block softened cream cheese
2 tbsp melted butter
1/4 tsp vanilla
1 package sugar-free cherry Jell-O

Directions
- Blend and pour into moulds/ice cube trays and freeze until solid
- Melt sugar-free chocolate chips in a double boiler
- Roll bombs in the chocolate
- Refrigerate to harden

Nutritional Information per fat bomb
87 calories
9 g fat
0.5 g carbohydrates
0 g fiber
1.5 g protein

Peanut Butter Balls

96 balls
Prep time: 30 mins
Total time: 90 mins

Balls
2 1/2 cups natural peanut butter
1 cup sweetener (depending on your desired level of sweetness)
3 cups nuts (chopped peanuts, pecans, and almonds)
3 cups unsweetened coconut
1/4 cup soft butter

Coating
5 oz (140 g) dark, sweetened chocolate (mix of 70% and Stevia sweetened chocolate)
1 square Baker's unsweetened chocolate
3/4 cup butter (instead of Parowax)
1 tbsp whipping cream

Directions
- Refrigerate balls before dipping
- The natural pb makes them a challenge to roll, so drop by spoonful

Dark Chocolate Mint Fat Bombs

12 fat bombs

Prep time: 20 mins
Total time: 2 hrs

1/4 cup coconut oil
4 tbsp butter
1/4 cup sweetener, or to taste
1/2-1 tsp peppermint extract
4 oz sugar-free dark chocolate, chopped
1 tbsp butter

Directions
- Line a muffin pan with 12 silicone or parchment liners, or use candy moulds
- Heat the coconut oil and butter until melted; add sweetener and peppermint extract
- Divide mixture among the cups/moulds and refrigerate again until set
- Melt together chocolate and butter in a double boiler or in a glass dish over simmering water
- Divide the chocolate mixture and spoon on top of the coconut oil/butter layer
- Refrigerate until set

Nutritional Information per fat bomb
125 calories
12 g fat
3 g carbohydrates
0.5 g fiber
0.5 g protein

Peanut Butter Fudge

Makes 15 pieces

Prep time: 30 mins
Total time: 2 hrs

1/2 cup butter
1/2 cup whipping cream
1 cup natural peanut butter
1 tsp vanilla extract
3/4 cup powdered sweetener (Swerve), or to taste
1/4 cup almond flour

Directions
- Line a 9x5" loaf pan with parchment paper
- In a medium saucepan over medium heat, bring the butter and cream to a boil; boil 2 mins
- Remove from heat; add peanut butter and vanilla extract
- Transfer to a large bowl; beat in powdered sweetener 1/2 cup at a time; mixture will begin to separate and become clumpy
- Mix in almond flour
- Press the mixture evenly into the prepared loaf pan and refrigerate until set, at least 1 hr
- Remove the parchment paper by the edges and cut the fudge into small squares

Nutritional Information per piece
190 calories
18 g fat
5 g carbohydrates
1.3 g fiber
4.5 g protein

Gingerbread Balls

Makes 12 balls

Prep time: 30 mins
Total time: 90 mins

2 cups almond flour
2/3 cup Swerve sweetener or Monk Fruit sweetener
1 teaspoon ground ginger
1/2 teaspoon ground cinnamon
1/2 teaspoon ground nutmeg
1/4 teaspoon salt
6 tablespoons melted butter

Directions
- In a medium-sized bowl mix dry ingredients until combined
- Stir in melted butter to form a thick dough
- Roll into balls
- Place the balls in an airtight container and refrigerate for 1 hr

Nutritional Information per ball
160 calories
15 g fat
4 g carbohydrates
2 g fiber
4 g protein

Sugar-free Eggnog

Makes 4 servings

Prep time: 30 mins
Total time: 90 mins

4 large eggs
2 large egg yolk
1/2 cup granular Swerve Sweetener (or 1/4 cup Swerve and 1/4 tsp liquid Stevia extract)
1/4 tsp salt
4 cups unsweetened almond milk
2 1/2 tsp vanilla extract, divided
1/2 tsp ground nutmeg
1/2 cup whipping cream
1 tbsp powdered Swerve sweetener

Directions
- In a large saucepan, combine eggs, yolks, sweetener, and salt
- Slowly whisk in milk until well combined
- Cook mixture over low heat while stirring constantly, until it becomes thick enough to coat the back of a spoon and registers 165° F (this can take up to 15 mins)
- Stir in 2 tsp vanilla and nutmeg and let cool
- Transfer to covered container and refrigerate
- Just before serving, whip cream with sweetener and remaining vanilla into soft peaks and gently fold into the egg mixture

Nutritional Information per serving
225 calories

...more

continued...

19.5 g fat
4 g carbohydrates
1.1 g fiber
9.2 g protein

Keto Stuffing
Makes 4 servings

Prep time: 15 mins
Total time: 45 mins

3 keto rolls
1 small onion, chopped
2 tbsp summer savoury
2 tbsp softened butter

Directions
- Break rolls in a food processor; add other ingredients and process, but not too finely
- Place in a covered casserole dish and bake at 350° F for 30 mins
- Adjust proportions and cooking time as you like for taste/quantity

Nutritional Information per serving
190 calories
15.5 g fat
7.5 g carbohydrates
4.5 g fiber
5.5 g protein

Cauliflower Mash
6 servings

Prep time: 30 mins
Total time: 45 mins

1 large head cauliflower, steamed soft
1 tub of Philadelphia whipped chives dip
1/2 cup butter
1 tbsp whipping cream
salt to taste

Directions
- Press water out of cooked cauliflower and mash well with remaining ingredients
- Serve hot

Nutritional Information per serving
270 calories
24 g fat
8 g carbohydrates
2 g fiber
5 g protein

Gravy

drippings from roasted meat
salt/spice to taste
1/2 tsp xanthan gum dissolved in 1 cup water

Directions
- Mix ingredients and bring to a boil until thickened

Cranberry Sauce

6 servings

Prep time: 20 mins
Total time: 90 mins

1 cup water
1 cup erythritol/Stevia sweetener or
other sweetener to taste
3 cups cranberries
1/2 tsp grated orange zest

Directions
- Bring water and sugar to a boil,
  stirring until sugar is dissolved
  Add cranberries and simmer,
  stirring occasionally, until berries
  just pop, 10-12 mins
- Stir in zest
- Cool before serving

Nutritional Information per serving
23 calories
0 g fat
3.5 g carbohydrates
1 g fiber
0 g protein

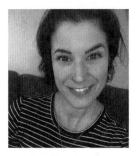

I started my Keto/LCHF journey in May 2017. I was suffering greatly with horrible insomnia to the point of seeing my doctor and trying medication, but having no success. I had heard of this "fad" diet Keto and how people were losing a lot of weight. I myself have never struggled with my weight as I'm very active and have an active job, but it piqued my interest so I started doing some research. In the research I had gone through books, the Internet, documentaries, and just talking to others who do this WOE (way of eating), and I learned it really isn't a new "diet." It's been around for a long time and it's us, as people, who have changed the way we eat/overeat.

I also learned in addition to weight loss there were so many benefits, and better sleep was one! I figured I had nothing to lose since I tried other things to help and it was really affecting my life and health, so I started that week. After three days of clean Keto and tracking my food (for my own knowledge) I slept all night—ALL night! I was thrilled and I felt pretty good so I decided to adopt this lifestyle. Within two weeks I was down 13 pounds, sleeping all night, and the residual back pain I had also dealt with from an issue stemming back years was virtually gone. This was a lovely addition because I had all but learned to just live with that pain. I have learned so much about this WOE and its benefits that it's all but a no-brainer to live and eat this way.

- Amber

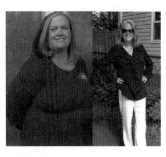

No one other than my husband has seen the picture on the left. It was October 8, 2016, and I was crushed when I saw that picture.

We had just spent an awesome weekend celebrating my 49th birthday. We saw Adele, a hockey game, the CN tower, and had reconnected with a childhood friend. On the night of my birthday, we went to Medieval Times and they took that picture on the way in. We had a fantastic evening and on the way out, they handed us that picture. I knew I was overweight, but really didn't see myself as this size

That night I vowed that by the time I hit 50, things were going to be different!! I turned 50 in 2017 and was well on my way to a healthier me. I am still a work in progress but I am NOT that person anymore!

It was extremely overwhelming in the beginning. I was 261 pounds wearing a 3X/22 pants. I had over 100 pounds to lose. I had mobility issues, self-esteem issues, and self-doubt. I had many people arguing that what I was doing couldn't be healthy. BUT I had all of you (Keto Solution Community)! I had my husband, my kids, and my parents cheering me on. I thank every single one of you for being here with me. xox

- Cathy

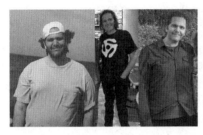

I started LCHF in September 2017. I've always struggled with weight and TRYing to eat correctly with no luck. Always finding it a constant struggle to lose weight. Always trying to lose other than just living and not worrying about it. I'm grateful for Angela's expertise in this area and she was able to confirm a lot of things I've been reading, watching, and researching.

My testimonial is the best thing I'm able to offer. I'm just tired of TRYing. Now I'm DOing. Keto may not be for everyone, but it sure is for me.

- David

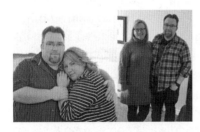

My husband and I live in PEI with our two daughters. We started LCHF/Keto May 30, 2017, and have been following this way of eating without a break ever since. I've always struggled with my weight and received a diagnosis of diabetes a month before starting Keto.

My husband and I dove right in and there's no looking back for us. Between the two of us, we've lost almost 200 pounds, I'm no longer diabetic, and our energy, mental clarity, and overall quality of life is so much better than before LCHF/Keto. We'll never go back to eating a high-carb diet. We can't. We were so unhealthy and unhappy. Keto Solution has been such an amazing support to us. It's helped us by providing a solid education in how this way of eating makes you healthier, how to eat LCHF/Keto in a healthy way, providing recipes and ideas, and providing support.

- Jill

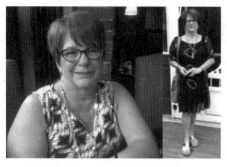

Keto has changed our lives! Ed and I are so grateful to those who have guided us on our Keto journey. Keto has given me freedom! Freedom from taking short-acting insulin with every meal — no more insulin with meals! Also, a major cutback on my long-acting insulin from 43 to 25 units! Plus a major drop in my AIC from 9.2 to 7.8 and a weight loss of 29 pounds that has given me back my youthful figure. Plus we both have more energy and I don't take my acid reflux medication anymore. Ed has reduced his thyroid medication and no more acid reflux. Keto is the way to go!

- Linda

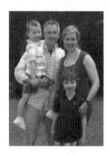

I am a Registered Nurse certified in Endoscopy, but have experience in many other hospital departments. I'm from Sydney, Cape Breton, where my parents are still living as well as my husband's family, too. I am an RCMP wife and have lived in many different provinces. We came to PEI from Nunavut, where we lived in Iqaluit for four years; and then we were posted to Summerside. We lived there for seven years and had two boys before moving to Stratford two years ago. We have also lived in the Rockies of Alberta and BC. I love to ski/snowboard, snowshoe, walk my big dog, and work out at home when I find the time. My weight has always fluctuated, but I have always been able to maintain a normal healthy weight. My parents are also healthy and active at ages 71 and 79; both are taking no medications. I had 10 pounds of extra weight to lose and exercise alone was not getting the results I wanted. I had been researching the Keto lifestyle for many months before applying it to my life and quickly shed the 10 pounds I was looking to lose. But then I was hooked. I loved the food, I loved not having food on my mind all day and was happier than I'd been in a while. My husband is also on board, but not as strict as me yet, which is fine. And my family and in-laws are also interested in learning about Keto and open to learning how to incorporate low carbs into their diets. I am so excited to have found this Keto family and want to be a part of the wonderful way you are spreading Keto goodness. I am in awe of all of your personal journeys with Keto: the benefits are so much more than weight loss! I can't wait to soak up your knowledge and support the group in any way that I can. Thank you for the opportunity. I will not let you down.

- Alison

Additional Resources

Websites
dietdoctor.com
carynzinn.com
ditchthecarbs.com
doctoraseem.com
thefatemperor.com
smashthefat.com
whatthefatbook.com
lchf-rd.com
healthfulpursuit.com
ketovangelistkitchen.com
burnfatnotsugar.com

Documentaries
- Fat Head (2009)
- Cereal Killers Movie (2013)
- Fat, A Documentary (2019)

Books
- *Simply Keto* by Suzanne Ryan
- *The New Atkins for a New You* by Dr. Eric C. Westman
- *The Art and Science of Low Carbohydrate Living* by Dr. Jeff S. Volek and Dr. Stephen D. Phinney
- *Eat Rich Live Long* by Dr. Ivor Cummins and Dr. Jeffry Gerber
- *The Big Fat Surprise* by Nina Teicholz
- *Lies My Doctor Told Me* by Dr. Ken D. Berry
- *The Obesity Code* by Dr. Jason Fung
- *The Diabetes Code* by Dr. Jason Fung
- *Diabetes Unpacked* by various authors (The Noakes Foundation)
- *The Pioppi Diet* by Dr. Aseem Malhotra and Donal O'Neill
- *The Diet Fix* by Dr. Zoë Harcombe
- *Good Calories Bad Calories* by Gary Taubes
- *Why We Get Fat* by Gary Taubes
- *Real Meal Revolution* by Tim Noakes, Jonno Proudfoot, and Sally-Ann Creed

Podcasts
- Low Carb MD Podcast
- The Obesity Code Podcast
- 2 Keto Dudes
- Diet Doctor Podcast with Dr. Bret Scher

YouTube Channels
- KenDBerryMD
- Dr. Richard K. Bernstein
- Low Carb Down Under

Organizations
- The Noakes Foundation
- Canadian Clinicians for Therapeutic Nutrition
- Public Health Collaboration (UK)
- Diabetes (UK)

Acknowledgements

I am so grateful to all those who contributed to this guide and cookbook, especially to my sister, Susan Howarth, who has been with me from the beginning, encouraging me and helping me with so much proofreading and editing suggestions. I also want to thank the Keto Solution Admin team, David Rashed, Codi Shewan, Jill Sabean, Stephanie Scharf, Alison Stanhope-Morrison, Gerry Fougere, my sister Carolyn Campbell, and Amber Jackson. Amber not only contributed many of the recipes, she also spent many hours collecting and organizing them. Also, a huge thank you to the members of the Keto Solution Facebook Group who contributed recipes: Gwendolyn Mullen, Jill Sabean, Gerry Fougere, and Linda Doiron, Finally, thanks to my wife, Nora McKenna, for all the encouragement and support over the last few years for me to follow my passion for Keto and helping others along their health journeys.

Index